The
Sixth Battle

The
Sixth Battle

A Story of Alzheimer's, Love, and Faith

By
Mary Lennon Koch

iUniverse, Inc.
Bloomington

The Sixth Battle
A Story of Alzheimer's, Love, and Faith

iUniverse books may be ordered through booksellers or by contacting:

iUniverse
1663 Liberty Drive
Bloomington, IN 47403
www.iuniverse.com
1-800-Authors (1-800-288-4677)

ISBN: 978-1-4759-7418-8 (sc)
ISBN: 978-1-4759-7420-1 (hc)
ISBN: 978-1-4759-7419-5 (ebk)

Library of Congress Control Number: 2013902151

Printed in the United States of America

iUniverse rev. date: 02/06/2013

Dedication

To Mom, for your faithful care for Dad.

To Ken, for finding the tools to help me get started, and for not resenting one minute of my time devoted to Dad or his story.

To Martha, for telling me for fourteen years, "You should be a writer . . . !"

To June, for your interest and support.

Table of Contents

Preface

This book is not a medical journal about Alzheimer's data but an observation of my father's death from Alzheimer's. My observation is wrapped in love, admiration, devotion, and detail in the hopes of giving flesh and blood to statistics and facts. It is largely my efforts to journal my father's life after his Alzheimer's diagnosis, but because of the age in which we live and how easy it is to communicate immediately through email, my mom, siblings, husband, and in-laws all contributed in some measure. I couldn't have done this love-project without any of them.

Well into Dad's disease, we participated in the Alzheimer's Memory Walk and were known as the Lennon Super Six. Our name came from Dad's division in World War II, the Super Sixth Armored Division, and because "we" were the six children of Mom and Dad. Super Six was a perfect fit. After all was said and done, though, there were not just six of us on the Memory Walk Team, but thirty-nine who walked out of love for Dad. As for his care, many more than the six children enlisted to help Dad and Mom while they suffered through Alzheimer's. I pray the same will be true for you, if you have a loved one fighting this disease.

A story is no good without facts, and even less without heart. When I was putting this memoir together, I wondered why I had fewer and fewer entries towards the end of Dad's life. His last year is hardly recorded. I went back through other journals not devoted to Dad and discovered that during his last year my family had its own turmoil that kept me from recording his story. It's an easy answer to the missing days and months. A less obvious answer is maybe it was God's mercy to spare me or anyone else having to re-live Dad's slow death, page after page. The suffering is mind-numbing. I cried almost as much for him while putting this book together, as I did any time all the days of his dying.

Memories

Say hello to my Dad, Horace Lennon. Don't talk loudly but do look him in the eye when you speak to him. Smile and shake his hand. He's been diagnosed with Alzheimer's and he's unnerved. We all are. It didn't take a diagnosis for us to suspect something was wrong. What was right with this man was that he was a man of faith and courage, both labels fully supported by his life. He was known as Horace Lennon to many people, but to us he was known as Dad. We were naive about what this diagnosis meant. We didn't realize he was headed off to war and the battle would be fought right in his own house this time. Although he escaped death a number of times in WWII, he never thought he would escape it completely. It wasn't death that had him unnerved. It was dying.

Two timepieces belonged to my dad. One was a Tri-Compac Watch, given by the Universal Watch Company of Geneva, Switzerland for the Swiss government. The other was a grandfather's clock given as a gift from his children for his seventieth birthday. His Tri-Compac watch and his grandfather's clock were dear to him. The one represented valor and the other represented love, and they book-ended the best years of his life, I think. Both of these timepieces no longer tell time because Dad broke them. Instead, they tell a story about a man diagnosed with Alzheimer's.

He came home from World War II with four medals and a watch from the Universal Watch Company of Geneva, Switzerland. The watch was inscribed with the words, "Presented to most worthy deserving soldier 6th Arm'd Div. Tech. Sgt. H. W. Lennon by Maj. Gen. R. W. Grow 23 June 1945." This "worthy deserving" soldier fought in five WWII battles: Normandy, Northern France, Ardennes,

Rhineland, and Central Europe, including the Battle of the Bulge. His four medals were the Bronze Star, the Silver Star, the Silver Star with Oak Leaf Cluster, and the Croix de Guerre (awarded by France). This soldier was my father, Horace Warrington Lennon, Sr.

The date was September 26, 1945. Dad was coming home. World War II was over. It was historically documented for its devastation, carnage, and number of lives lost. Shamefully understated, men fought and died in that war, or fought and came home to live with their memories. Daddy was one of the fortunate ones who came home with his memories to the love of a seventeen-year-old girl named Lillian Dorine (Pat to her family). Besides the medals on his chest and the watch on his arm, he wanted a kiss on his lips from that seventeen-year-old girl.

He was from Delco, NC. She was originally from the state of New York, and a more unlikely pair you can't imagine. He was rural. She was urban. He was the son of a tobacco farmer. She was the daughter of a pastor and an educator. He was twenty-six and had been overseas. She was seventeen and had only read about overseas from his letters. Yet Providence brought them together as Providence does through a series of events that ended up in a little country church in Livingston, NC, halfway between her parents' home in Lake Waccamaw and the tobacco fields of Delco. Her father was the pastor of the church. His father was the chairman of the deacons. Horace and Pat had only met once when he came home for a short furlough before being deployed overseas. From that one-time encounter, they courted by mail for more than two years.

His homecoming day was hot, humid, partly cloudy, and the most glorious day in almost three years. Pat was beside herself at seeing Horace. The first and only time they met before he left for war, she was fifteen years old. He was twenty-four, and he was considered the county's most eligible bachelor. Their romance budded and blossomed through the US Mail, but now time and distance would no longer keep them apart. They would be face to face again after twenty-seven months. The US Mail had brought word from Horace that the first thing he wanted when he got home was a kiss. What was she going to do? She'd never kissed a man before! On September 26th, his car turned down her street, while she turned and ran, hiding behind her family's woodpile. It would buy her some time to think. Buddy, her dog, thought she was playing Hide and Seek, so he barked, "I found you!" Mortified that a soldier who hadn't run from combat might find her crouched behind a woodpile, she jumped up and ran back into the house. He was there, tall, tan, fit, and waiting for his kiss. They were married two months later, November 25, 1945, just weeks after her eighteenth birthday.

During the next twenty-five years, Daddy managed an auto parts store in the county seat of Whiteville, NC. He was also ordained as a minister of the gospel and pastored a small church in the Delco area. He had a reputation as a man of character, able to do hard things but gentle in his dealings with people. His parents and Mama's father died. Six children were born. After twenty-five years in Whiteville, he felt led to be a part of the Christian school movement. He uprooted his family, moving them to Goldsboro, NC, where he went to work for Goldsboro Christian Schools. When we moved, the *Whiteville News Reporter* wrote this about him: "To describe Horace Lennon to a community which has known him for 25 years is perhaps unnecessary, but—He is a man of moral strength; he is a man of unswerving faith. Horace Lennon has moved about Whiteville with a quiet dignity, with never an exchange of conviction for the sake of expediency. He bows his head before God, and remains upright and erect before men." [1]

Daddy was the business manager for Goldsboro Christian Schools for one year when the school's mechanic left. Twenty-seven buses sat on the grounds without anyone to maintain them. Daddy traded in his suit for mechanic's overalls at the request of school leadership and kept the fleet of buses running. Since he had tested as a mechanical genius in the army, he was a logical choice for this job. However, this is not how we envision our lives progressing, from medals to community accolades to bus mechanic. He worked under hard conditions for eleven years. He never complained or whined and never updated his resume "because he deserved better." He knew the principle of contentment and godliness. Eventually, the school terminated his employment and he and Mama moved to Greenville, SC, where most of their children lived.

---

[1]   *Whiteville News Reporter*, "A 25 Year Sojourn," 18 Feb 1971, sec. B2.

In Greenville, Daddy became a self-employed carpenter. Mama provided daycare services for their grandchildren. They were active in their church and God gave them wonderful friends. They loved their neighbors as themselves. Most important was their influence in the lives of their children, grandchildren, and great grandchildren.

Sadly, you aren't meeting Daddy at his best, when he was pinned with a medal, or cited for bravery in a battle, or when he served a ministry, or provided for and loved his family. You're meeting him during the most difficult time of his life, his battle with Alzheimer's.

Diagnosis: Alzheimer's

"Something's not right. I want Daddy to go for a checkup." Mom had observed some stark inconsistencies with Dad. He seemed unable to tell time, and he forgot that their neighbor died. He was supposed to pray at the funeral! The doctor did a thorough physical, ruled out other possibilities without extreme measures like CAT scans or MRI's, and did the infamous Alzheimer's test. Simple questions, pictures, and activities if your brain is working right. A bright spotlight equal to the Inquisition, if it's not. The doctor was very kind, but he confirmed based on the test results that Daddy had Alzheimer's. One of the tests was the ability to draw a clock face and record the correct time. Dad was unable to do this. A timepiece no longer spoke of valor or love, but rather of mortality.

Shock. Fear. Sorrow. Depression. Those were some of the emotions we experienced as well as Daddy. None of us knew how to handle the news. Dad knew the doctor had delivered a terminal diagnosis but Alzheimer's was already robbing him of complete comprehension. Sometime later, I stayed with him while Mama took a break. It was a rainy, chilly day. We sat together on the couch in the darkness, which added to his depression and wasn't very wise on my part. He began talking slowly about his health. He knew something was wrong, but wasn't sure what it was.

I remember being surprised at how devastated he appeared to be that he had been diagnosed with a terminal illness. Now, I'm surprised at my insensitivity, but before you judge me too harshly, I must tell you that Dad was a man with an unshakable faith in an unshakable God. He trusted the eternal keeping of his soul in the saving act of Jesus' death on the cross and had devoted a lifetime to telling others about the saving grace of God. His Christianity was so tightly woven through all of his daily activities, that his life *was* full-time Christian service. It didn't matter if he was a deacon at his church or putting the finishing touches on cabinetry or fighting a war, his life was not different based on his surroundings.

He had often said, "When I'm no longer able to work, I pray that God will just take me home!" He shed tears over dead parents, over dead brothers and sisters, and talked of seeing them again. He cried with me over the death of one of my daughters. He had a desire to see his Lord and his family again, so his attitude was new to me. I'm ashamed to admit that I never stopped to consider how important life is to a person until it's ending. He did not lose his faith and suddenly question the reality of heaven or his salvation. Nor did he question the existence of God or what He was going to accomplish. However, I believe the Bible is very clear that there can be intense times of darkness for the soul of a Christian, and that's what happened to Daddy.

He sat on the couch looking out the window. "I don't know what's wrong with me . . . it's something that's not good . . . not good. I know . . . I think I have something wrong that will take my life. I'm not sure how much time I have." And with that, he started crying. I cried too.

"Daddy," I put my arm around him. "Daddy, you have Alzheimer's. I don't know if you remember the doctor talking about it or not. It affects your mind and yes, if the Lord tarries, it will be the end of you, but you have years ahead of you before that happens." Looking back, they were such foolish words. While Dad had just been diagnosed, Alzheimer's was already at work making it difficult for him to process. Besides, having your mortality confirmed is serious business.

Four and a half years into Dad's Alzheimer's, Mom recorded these words in early August 2002.

> *"Yesterday Daddy asked me several times if my mother and daddy were still living. Each time I told him no. The last time when I told him he started crying. I don't know how many of you know it, but Grandfather dropped dead in the bathroom and Daddy caught him. And of course, you all know the*

circumstances about Mudder. He has no memory of it. I didn't ask him; I could just tell.

This morning he said, 'Mary [his sister was named Mary], both your parents are still living, aren't they?' I hesitated. I didn't know whether to answer him as Mary or as me. Finally, I just quietly said, 'No.' He seemed surprised, then said, 'They're the same as mine?' A couple of weeks ago he had asked me about his parents. He wondered where they were and why he never saw them."

Later that same month, August 20th turned out to be a special day in the world of Alzheimer's. When we headed to the pool where Mom exercised to pick her up, Dad said, "You know, I used to know people, know how to do things, remember stuff, but this Altimer's really takes it away from you." I don't think he had spoken that plainly about his disease before. I was amazed at how clear his mind seemed that day, even though his body seemed frailer. I told him I pray for him every day because I knew it was tough. He cried.

I didn't know it then, but every day was more precious than the one that came after it. His life was being taken from us and from him, sometimes slowly and other times at an alarming speed. Alzheimer's is not predictable.

Summer turned to fall, and already precious days were being replaced with nightmare days. In November, Dad got a stomach virus. Seven of us ended up contributing to his care during that time. That number was made up of children and in-laws, grandchildren, and even the fiancé of a grandchild. No one was exempt from helping and some were not exempt from catching the virus including Mom, who ended up in the hospital for a day. The virus attack was just days before Mom's and Dad's 57th anniversary.

With Alzheimer's, there are occasionally roses among the thorns. I had bought Mom and Dad cards for each to give to the other. Sunday, on the way to church, we stopped by their house to drop off the cards for their anniversary the next day. I ran in the house and hurriedly told Daddy he should sign the card and give it to Mama. Then I left them in the bedroom having family devotions.

I put the card at his place at the table, and wrote a hasty note on a napkin. It said, "Dear Daddy, you can sign this card for Mama with something like
'Love, Horace'"

and I signed it "Love, Mary."

Later, as I was thinking about Dad and the card, I grew concerned that something might happen to the card, that he might see it and get confused, or that he might even throw the napkin away and give the card to Mom unsigned. I called and Dad answered the phone. I talked to him about the card, telling him that I had put it on the table with a napkin and that I had written an explanation. He sounded confused but said thanks. I asked him did he want me to come over in the morning and help him sign it, and he said yes. I could tell he was distracted. I asked him what was going on and he said, "I'm waiting for some woman to come help my wife." I said, "Oh? Is something wrong? I think Kaaren's coming over." He said, "Yes! Kaaren, that's who." Then he gave the phone to Mama.

Her recovery from the virus had been remarkable aided by IV fluids. Once she was home though, her condition deteriorated rapidly. She had asked Dad for juice but he couldn't bring it to her. He was heartbroken because he knew he couldn't help her even in that small way.

We went straight to the house and, along with Kaaren, got things mildly under control. Then Mama showed me the card. It was beautiful and very touching because he had done it all by himself. A rose moment buried in the thorns.

He had signed it:

Love alway   to you-
   Horace   Pat
(on the envelope)

Love for my wife
             Horace_
(inside the card)

2003 — Giving Up Ground

The Best Day of the Year

Daddy helped me with the Christmas decorations on January 2nd. He was proud and happy to help while I was worried and anxious! Taking down the decorations at Mom's and Dad's house involved a 6-foot tree, attic stairs, boxes, hundreds of lights, garland, and breakable ornaments and decorations.

He was unsure how to navigate the stairs, hold onto the railing, and transport boxes. I watched him analyze the physics of the matter the best way he could, figuring out fulcrum, leverage, support, etc. On the one hand, he did well with lots of determination and success. On the other hand, it was sad because physics was a language he knew by heart. The only way I can compare it is to someone who plays the piano by ear rather than by the skill of reading music. I don't think Dad could give you equations, but he knew by "ear" just what needed to be done to move, to fit, to reach point B from point A, to lift, to fix. I took his genius for granted when I was younger, assuming those skills came to everyone when they arrived at his age. It doesn't!

I was scared he was going to fall off the attic ladder and get hurt. I prayed God would keep him safe, and allow him to successfully complete what he had started. I had taken empty (easy) boxes down. Dad put the filled, heavy boxes up. There were two garland boxes, one box of ornaments that got tossed somewhere we'll never see again! and a box of lights that was awkward to navigate. While he was on the ladder, I wondered if Mama was disgusted because she thought I was thinking, *Look at my dad! He's very capable. Not at all like you make him out to be.* I wasn't thinking that, though. I was thinking two things: *God, please protect my dad!* and *I don't want to have to tell my sisters and brother he got hurt!* (because it looked like a done deal).

After we put the decorations up in the attic, I pulled the Christmas tree box towards him so he could get it down. That box just doesn't like to go up or down their attic; I was sure he would lose his footing. He was uncertain but determined, and I was glad. He was able to carry it all the way to the living room where the tree was waiting for us. Dad paid close attention to how I removed the branches. "Is that all there is to it?" he asked after watching me remove a few branches. I said, "Yep!" And he helped me take down the entire tree. When a branch got stuck, he would tell me, "You let me get that one. You just have to give it the shock treatment . . . a yank! and it comes" while he demonstrated the whole thing to me with a grab and yank. So that's how we did it. When one branch would be stubborn, I would leave it for him. He would stop where he was working and get it out for me. He worked hard and at a good speed in spite of random confusion. Sometimes, when one of his branches became stuck, he would try to unscrew the trunk. We managed to get the whole tree down and back up in the attic without any events.

A couple of times, Daddy said, "Thank you so much! I'm so glad you let me help." One time he said, "I've felt useful today!" I told him he was far more useful than taking down a Christmas tree. I hoped all the lifting and stair climbing didn't cause him to have a bad night's sleep that night. I asked God to give him and Mama good, wonderful sleep the entire night through.

Looking back, January 2, 2003 was the best day of the year.

Understanding the Situation

Sometime in the last half of 2002, the grandfather's clock stopped working. Dad loved that clock. He was meticulous with his and Mama's possessions, with their home, their cars, anything and everything. He had lived through the Depression. During his pre-teen years, the price of farmland fell 50%. Circumstances could rob you of half of your assets overnight. Laziness and carelessness could take the other 50% in almost the same amount of time. Yet, it wasn't the value of the possessions or the possessions themselves that made him take care of them, but the principle of good stewardship. He was a steward of the things God had given him, so even a broken grandfather's clock would weigh on him. Mom called a repairman after the clock stopped working the first time. He was called back several times, either because he didn't fix the clock, or he fixed it poorly, or Dad over-wound it. Finally, the repairman got the clock working consistently.

From time to time, Dad tried to wind the clock again. For every one of his attempts, Mama would tell him to leave it alone because of all they had been through getting it repaired. This frustrated Dad. One day, Mama found Daddy in the living room messing with the clock again. "Honey, leave the clock alone! The repairman just got it working right after all these months. Please leave it alone!" She took the cabinet key from him. He responded by hitting her in the chest! My dad hit my mom! I never saw this man do anything hurtful with his hands, towards my mom or any other human, or even our animals. He had combat training but his hands didn't naturally harm *anything*. When Mama was recounting the story, she said it hurt. I can only imagine. At this point in the disease, he experienced childish emotions and lack of control, but there was nothing childish about his strength.

Mama gave Daddy the key. "It's your clock. You do whatever you want to with it," she said. Over the course of the next month, he messed and messed with it, and she left him alone. I'm sure it was difficult to watch him tear up something that was so dear. No one knows exactly when he broke the grandfather's clock. Its silence gave testimony to the sadness of Alzheimer's, and it brought to light his violence against Mom.

The week of January 9, 2003, Daddy messed with the clock again. He thought the door was broken because he couldn't remember how to lock it. "Some . . . someone's . . . broken this uh . . . uhhm . . ." He fumbled for words and with the cabinet door, trying to re-lock it. "No, honey. It just needs to be locked." Blank stare. "What? What did you say?" Dad asked. "It just needs to be locked." "Will you come show me?" Now, Mom was afraid. If she tried to show him and he got angry, he might hit her again. Kindness and courage prevailed, and she showed him how to lock the cabinet door.

Suddenly, Dad started crying and said, "I've . . . forgotten how. I've forgotten . . . how . . . to take care of my clock . . . and I'm . . . I'm tearing it up." He looked at Mama. "Don't let me do that, okay?" pleading through his tears.

"The last time I tried to stop you, you hit me." Mom said with a touch of fear and a quiet, breaking heart.

A bomb of sorrow went off in Dad's heart. Tears. Apologies. Repentance. He was crushed and maybe a little disbelieving because he couldn't remember. He was a man with four medals. He fought in five battles. Had citation after citation for bravery and honor. He had six children who loved and respected him. He was asked to be the mayor of a town where they had lived. He was an ordained minister. More than all of these, he loved his wife. He would never intentionally hurt her.

As a family we talked about it on a conference call, believe it or not, even though we all lived in the same city. We discussed what we had observed, we talked through this new situation, and we tried to make sense between reality and diagnosis. The caregiver suffers like no one else. Caring for someone while grieving for them takes a mental and physical toll. Dad's lost-ness and mistakes, his mood swings and inabilities brought hourly surprises. Common sense tried to control and correct those things but it was useless. Alzheimer's robbed him of ability and understanding, yet at times he understood enough to feel shame and humiliation over what he'd done. Daddy got smaller and smaller, more and more unsure of his movements or activities. It was pitiful to watch. Mom's health was going downhill. The doctor had told us that consistency slows down the progression of Alzheimer's, and consistency became Mom's focus and her gift to Dad. She guarded his routine like it was some treasure, and it was. How could we treat that faithfulness as a virtue to be cast aside? What could we do that would help with Dad's care and give her some relief, too?

From that phone call, we agreed on three things. Mom and Dad needed help now. Mom and Dad needed ongoing, regular help. We needed a plan for dealing with emergencies. Nothing can prepare you for the time and resources it takes to care for someone with Alzheimer's, or the emotional and physical beating that comes with it. There are six of us children. Before it was all over, we experienced every range of emotions, from wishing there were twelve of us to wishing we could divorce each other like husbands and wives do. ("She's my ex-sister" is a ridiculous statement, but heartache and grief can work extreme responses.) Thankfully, God brought us through.

Warren and June handled the immediate need. A couple of days after our conference call, Dad went for a visit to Warren's and Dawn's house five blocks from our parents' home while June picked Mom up from her exercise class at the local university's pool. She and Mom were able to talk while Dad was out of the house. It was an enlightening conversation, so much so, that while this book is about Dad's battle, her experience as his caregiver is a story of its own. He lived his dying days with amazing grace, and she loved him "for better, for worse, in sickness and in health, until death do us part."

Constant communication between Mom and the family became the norm in the early days of 2003. From that point on, Mom emailed the family as a group rather than singling out one child or another.

Thankfully, she was already familiar with email. Email could broadcast to all at the same time, and whoever was available first could respond. For emergencies, we came up with a decision tree. We had three blessings that many families don't have: the number of siblings, that we all got along, and the proximity of our homes. Our decision tree looked like this.

We established a call chain. Birth order was easiest. Whoever Mom called, that person called the next in birth order.

A situation arose. Mama called or emailed someone right away before details got fuzzy.

Did Mama think it was an emergency?

Did the family think it was an emergency?

If Mama said yes, it was an emergency, we used Plan A below.

If Mama and family said no, no emergency existed, we used Plan B below.

If Mama and family disagreed (mainly Mama said no, but Family said yes), seek expert opinion.

Plan A:

The person who received the phone call immediately called the next in line using the call chain.

Person #1 called doctor.

Someone physically checked on Mama/Daddy

Someone prepared to stay with them until the family knew how to handle the situation based on the doctor's comments.

Plan B:

The person who received the phone call immediately called the next in line using the call chain.

Person #1 called doctor.

Someone kept the family updated on events through email (most likely Person #1, or someone Person #1 had relayed information to).

All of the families tried to schedule a few minutes with Mom and Dad, whether a meal or a brief visit, anything.

Tooth Trouble

While we were being enlisted into Dad's battle, Dad had his own troubles not caused by Alzheimer's but complicated by Alzheimer's. He was eighty-three and he had age-related health issues normal for seniors. This time, it was a tooth. While we were discovering the extent of Dad's decline, it became apparent that he had a tooth that bothered him. Sadly, with Alzheimer's, we often never knew if something was really wrong/hurting or if Dad was just confused. Add to the mix that hurting teeth could be a sign of imminent heart problems, and we suddenly had a serious situation.

June made a dentist's appointment for Dad. Dr. Healey was able to find the bad tooth in spite of Dad's inability to communicate the right tooth. Apparently Dad had been in real pain for some time. The tooth was bad enough that Dr. Healey sent him to the dental surgeon to have it pulled that same day.

It makes me sad to think that Dad was hurting . . . hurt for how long? . . . and was unable to communicate that to anyone. Times like this made me wonder just how far into this gig we were. How could a heart keep pumping and lungs keep breathing in such misery? Not tooth misery. Unable to understand what's happening misery and unable to communicate that *anything* is wrong misery. He never complained to me about it, but I'm not sure what I would have done if he had. Can you imagine what it would be like to hurt constantly, but not be able to communicate that to someone? Could you live like that and remain decent and somewhat polite? I couldn't.

Lassie, Hurricanes, and Alzheimer's

D addy was watching *Lassie Come Home* on TV. He was trying to tell me about it and all he could think to say was, "We have *Lassie Come Home* on the radio, and it's deee . . . deee-licious!"

The same summer that Dad found Lassie delicious became a summer of setting a record weather-wise. Summertime is notorious for hurricanes in the South and 2003 did not disappoint. There were sixteen named storms that year. The first storm of the year began six weeks before hurricane season's official beginning and the last two storms formed in December, after the official end of hurricane season. It was the longest hurricane season since 1952. [2]

So, what does weather have to do with Alzheimer's? I did not conduct a scientific experiment but I did observe that as each storm gathered intensity and tracked our way, Dad seemed affected. Medically, the connection was probably that bad weather affected arthritis, sinus, and vertigo, while Alzheimer's affected understanding and communication. Dad would recover some ground after each storm abated, but never, it seemed, as much as he had lost. Maybe it was because of the number of storms coming through and maybe it was just the nature of Alzheimer's.

---

[2]   NOAA National Climatic Data Center, State of the Climate: Hurricanes & Tropical Storms for Annual 2003, published online December 2003, retrieved February 16, 2012 from http://www.ncdc.noaa.gov/sotc/tropical-cyclones/2003/13.

The Village

It was so easy to ignore Daddy in conversation. Talking to him required that you slow down, break down complex thoughts into simpler ones, or drop them altogether. In order to keep pace with our fast tempo lives, it became easier to drop him out of the conversation. He seemed glad when this happened because he sensed we weren't talking to him. He knew Mama had someone to talk to, first of all, and second, he knew he didn't have to comprehend and/or respond to what was said.

One Saturday in August, I was cutting their grass and the girls were in the yard with plastic bags, trying to catch bugs for Abby's insect collection. It was not an abnormal day. When I got closer to the girls with the lawn mower, Lauren yelled, "Mama! Granddaddy's in the garage [*where all the chemicals, power tools, hammers, you name it, are*]. Do you think that's okay?" I was caught off guard for a minute. I said yes, it was probably fine because the power had been disconnected and all the tools were unplugged. She seemed satisfied.

This incident struck me two ways. Number one, caring for and watching an Alzheimer's person was a huge responsibility. We couldn't take our eyes off of him for a minute. The stress of that took a tremendous toll. He forgot what behaviors were dangerous, inconvenient, or downright unsociable, and when those actions were exhibited, we were caught off guard. The behaviors happened when we least expected them and they either embarrassed or caused danger. There wasn't any consistency to the patterns, and tomorrow could be different with very few incidents.

Number two, I realized how important it was to incorporate everyone into the team. I'm talking about a quality-of-life team; a safety team; a relief-for-the-caregiver team. We utilized everyone available: siblings, grandchildren, girlfriends, boyfriends, and in-laws, and made the biggest tag team possible.

The youngest grandchild in our clan was thirteen so no one was exempt. My parents loved to watch *Andy Griffith*, *Lassie*, *The Waltons*, etc. One time my youngest child was responsible for Dad, even though it was only for thirty or forty-five minutes. I told her, "The best thing you can do is turn on the TV and find one of those shows. He loves them, and will sit and watch it with you. That should be safe enough." Thankfully, my suggestion worked.

Observations and Garage Girl

D ad had lost his ability to use a fork and knife. Some days were worse than others. One day, he would pick most of his food up with his fingers and eat. Other days he'd pick his fork up from his plate where I'd laid it in his line of vision filled with food. He might hold the fork and even push it around the plate, but if he was successful with it, it was an accident. I couldn't remember when he stopped being able to use a fork and knife together. Anything that needed cutting, we chopped up in little manageable pieces for him.

When Dad took an aptitude test in the army, he scored as a mechanical genius. He loved carpentry. He always had a workshop full of power tools. He loved working with automobiles. He was the basic provider in every way for his wife and children. Even when we were grown and had left home, he helped us with major car repairs at first, then minor car repairs, and all types of home repairs. All the while he worked as a self-employed carpenter. His workshop had a variety of tools, tools for cars, woodworking, general home repairs, etc.

If you walked in the door and asked him a question about your car or your house, the first thing he did was to grab the key to his workshop and say something like, "Let's go see what I have." The workshop was his domain. The kitchen was my mom's. They were very traditional in their approach, but they fit together perfectly like a hand in a glove.

Imagine a dad and a mom so defined by these two differences. Mama was synonymous with being a homemaker. Daddy was synonymous with the provider and caretaker. His workshop supported this calling. Even though my dad had been diagnosed with Alzheimer's for five years, he would still go outside to the workshop with us to check over the lawn mower, putter around, look at his tools, and just generally be where he loved to be.

Just when I thought I had handled all things Alzheimer's, a new change happened. I was not prepared the first time I needed help in the garage and my mom went with me, while my dad made no effort to get up off the couch.

Commended, Confused

O ne morning in early September, Mom put the *God Bless America* CD on for Dad and then went to their bedroom to clean some spots off the mattress before putting on clean sheets. Because the spot treatment left the mattress wet, she went in search of the blow dryer. Dad was at the round table in the living room with a pitiful expression on his face, when Mom realized the CD had finished. She said, "Oh, your music has stopped. I'll put on some more for you." Dad began to cry. "Somebody . . . some uhhh . . . yelled at me." (Softly) "Said I was no good . . . not needed any more." Dad couldn't tell her if it was a man or woman or anything about the person but the verdict hurled against him crushed him. Fear is contagious and even though Mom knew no one else was in the house, the reality of his devastation couldn't be ignored. She wanted to call for help but couldn't get to a phone without leaving him. True love stayed with the wounded and calmed him down.

Whether this was a nightmare (he often fell asleep while sitting) or a hallucination, the effect was the same. Dad became troubled about his worthlessness and inability. Troubled but not vocal. He never was a man to dwell on himself, so the behavior we started seeing next was confusing at first.

His watch was proof he wasn't always confused and unable. More and more, he would finger the watch, look at it on his arm, turn it over so the inscription was showing, and ask Mom to read it. Then he began asking other people, family and friends, to look at his watch and read the inscription. We were *happy* to do this. It was a reminder of better days. The watch validated skill, wisdom, ability, and recognition by his peers and superiors.

Just three days after the CD incident, before lunch, he had asked Mom for the fifth time to read his watch. Then he said, "I . . . uh-h-h . . . I want you to have this engraved on . . . on . . . on . . . what do you engrave things on?" Mom replied that any number of things can be engraved. Then Dad said, "I want you to have it engraved here . . . on . . . my watch." Mom said, "Well, it's already on your watch. That's why you can read it." So confused. So sad.

One time in the grocery store, he showed the watch to a perfect stranger and asked her to read it. If we could have been present when he was awarded that watch, we'd have been proud to stand beside him. With Alzheimer's, when he interrupted a shopper to look at his watch, we were uncomfortable standing beside him. From proud to embarrassed. As hard as it was, our situation was nothing compared to his. He was dying.

Ten days later, Daddy had a big mess that soaked all the way through his jeans. As he was getting dressed after Mom had cleaned him up, he handed his watch to her and said, "Hon, there's . . . uh . . . something . . . on the back of this . . . see what it says." Mom said, "Do you want me to read it to you?" "Yes." Mom read these words again: "Presented to most worthy deserving soldier 6th Arm'd Div. Tech. Sgt. H. W. Lennon by Maj. Gen. R. W. Grow 23 June 1945." Dad said quietly, "You read it just right." Mom said to him, "And the right man got it, too."

Dad's response? "Thank you. I'm just . . . uh . . . having troubles now, huh?"

Days later, messed up jeans would have been called a good day. Panic. Unable to breathe and unable to think. Dad was nowhere to be found. Mom called Warren, beside herself with anguish and worry. Thankfully, Warren lived only one street away, so he drove around a couple of streets looking for Dad. A jogger was out running and Warren inquired whether he had seen Dad, but no Dad. He drove by the house a second time, and Dad and Mom were sitting on the front porch. Had Dad found his way back home?

As it was, Dad had never left home. He had been in the bathroom with the light off and wouldn't answer when mom called. He said he didn't hear. These stresses took their toll on her.

Warren stayed at the house and visited until Mom calmed down. These were the events of September 25, 2003, in a little neighborhood in Taylors, South Carolina, while the rest of the world went about its normal business. Disaster was averted at least one more time.

One Trip, Two Stories

The church had a men's retreat at a camp a short distance into the mountains, and Warren and Dad went. Warren recorded the weekend for the rest of us, and Mom recorded Dad's version. The two stories give some insight into the burden of the caregiver and into a mind with Alzheimer's.

Warren's version.

Dad and I left Mom's and Dad's house about 5:00 p.m. on Friday. Two men whom Dad was familiar with rode with us. The trip to the retreat was uneventful even though the drive took us up a winding, steep road. We got settled in our room about 6:45 or so. We were in the main lodge where the meetings were also held. Supper was at 7:30. Dad ate well and again there were no incidents. The evening service was from 8:30 to 9:30. I worried that Dad might go to sleep during the service, but he was alert the entire time, not dozing once. After the service, we headed straight back to our room and went to bed.

The next morning, Dad and I got up about 6:45 and I had Dad get in the shower first. I laid out some of his clothes while he was in the shower. When he had showered, I got him started dressing and then I jumped in the shower. Dad was completely dressed by the time I got out of the shower. There was one caveat. He had gotten into my suitcase and put on some of my clothes! We laughed over that and got the right clothes on Dad. Dad asked me what my name was. "My name is Warren." Dad said, "My name is Horace Warren." I told him we shared names because I was his son. Dad smiled at that.

After the morning service, we had free time. I took Dad to the target range and he got eight bull's eyes out of about 20 shots from 50 feet. It was amazing considering his one bad eye and his other not-so-great eye. Afterward, we ate lunch and had the afternoon service. We were on the way home by 4:30 Saturday afternoon.

Mom and Dad had a grand reunion when we got home. I dropped Dad off and went home myself. About 9:00 p.m., I went back over to their house to help with the bedtime routine and Mom was crying. I asked if she wanted to talk. She said she hadn't been very patient with Dad so I didn't press the issue. Dad kept telling Mom he was sorry for leaving her for eight weeks and he knew it must have been hard on her.

This trip helped me realize that Dad is a major full time responsibility. We had no major incidents while we were gone, but his care was still a full time responsibility. I felt like I never had any free time. I was watching to make sure he didn't fall, that he did take his pills, didn't get lost, didn't do something that would hurt him, etc. It was an exhausting 24 hours. It doesn't seem possible that it was barely more than 24 hours.

Dad's version of the story, recorded by Mom:

Dad and Warren were at the retreat different lengths of time when he tells about the weekend. Sometimes they were there a week, sometimes eight weeks, and sometimes everything in between. There were "thousands" of men there. The only time he gave a definite figure, it was about 5,000 men. Dad also referred to the "going" in terms of all the men "being taken." He must have been confused with being shipped here and there in the army. He also thought there were five men in the room where

he slept. Dad was telling me some of the remarks the men made
over his ability to shoot. I [Mom] asked him, "The men up at
The Wilds [the retreat facility]?" He said, "No." Then I asked,
"You mean in the Army?" He said, "Yes . . . They couldn't get
over it." I had heard men comment at the Super Sixth reunions
about what a shooter he was. The two experiences sort of melded
together in his mind.

When he put his watch on the morning after returning home, he asked Mom, "Have . . . have I ever told you the h-h-history of this?" She said, "Maybe. Tell me again and let's see." (Such love!) He said, "Well . . . it's written on the . . . uh back . . . but I can't read it."

State of Confusion

Routine was the Alzheimer's sufferer's greatest friend. The retreat robbed Dad of his routine and gave Alzheimer's more of him.

Mom and Dad often watched *Little House on the Prairie* while eating supper. Just a couple of days after Dad returned home, they were a few minutes later eating than their normal dinner time. Mom turned on the TV so they could see the beginning of the show while she put supper on the table. The Olsons (the storekeeper and his wife) were arguing and Mrs. Olson threatened to leave Mr. Olson. Mom turned the TV off so she could read the Bible verse before dinner and so Daddy could ask the blessing. He prayed earnestly for the Olsons and asked the Lord to help him and Mom know if there was any way he and Mom could help them. Such a tender heart. This was my Dad. He was concerned for others in spite of his own troubles.

Days later, Dad initiated this conversation with Mom, still suffering from the change in his routine.

Dad: "I'm ashamed to say it but I . . . uh . . . don't think I know my name and . . . I don't know . . . your name."

Mom: "Well, you say you *think* you don't know your name. Try. What's your name?"

Dad: (very slowly and hesitantly) "Horace . . . Warrington . . . Lennon."

Mom: (excited) "That's right! Good for you!"

Dad: "But who are you? I-I-I . . . uh . . . don't . . . know your name. What's your name?"

Mom: "Do you want my real name or the name you call me by?"

Dad: "Your real name."

Mom: "Lillian . . . Dorine . . . Lennon."

Dad: (A moment of understanding lit up his face. Then he sat
         bolt upright and shouted) "Praise the Lord! Praise the Lord!
         You've got the same last name that I have!"

Mom: (smiling) "I know. You gave it to me. You gave it to me
         when we got married."

Dad: "We got married?"

Mom: "Yes, we got married."

Dad: "Lillian Dorine, you're a . . . beautiful lady."

Mom: "Do you want to know the name you call me by?"

Dad: "Yes."

Mom: "Pat. You call me Pat. Everybody calls me Pat."

Dad: "Lillian Dorine, you're a . . . beautiful lady."

"Pat" was Mom's nickname and she preferred it over her real
name. Mom said Dad called her Lillian Dorine for about the next
hour and she wished that was something he *would* forget!

Is it 2003 or 1945 or 1920? Yes.

Yesterday the girls and I stopped by Mama's and Daddy's house after shopping. Daddy sat in the living room. Mama was cooking. I went into the living room and said hello to him. He was talking to Lauren, and looked much the same as usual. More and more he asked outright "who's this?" or "who's that coming in here?" The calendar said it was 2003, but it might as well have been 1947 before any of his children were born.

I sat down beside him on the piano bench, maybe a foot or two away. I noticed he and Mama were both bundled up with sweaters and looked like they were ready for a snowstorm. Truthfully, the house was cold. It hadn't warmed up yet even though it was 3:00 in the afternoon.

His hands were cold. I took one of them in my hands to warm it up. He had a pillow on the recliner foot rest, and he was telling Lauren about something that had just happened. He said, "You know, I don't know how long it's been like this . . ." and he looked around and fumbled with the recliner lever. "I don't know how long it's been like this . . . that I didn't know how this . . ." and he trailed off. Was he trying to tell us that he was sitting in the chair and had wanted to get up, but couldn't remember how to operate the lever? I didn't know.

Later, I found out he tried to get up but he fell. He called Mama to come help him because he didn't know how to get out of the chair. He had tried on his own, couldn't figure it out, and got his one leg stuck in between the footrest and the chair itself. At this point, he called Mama.

She found him with one leg trapped in the opening. Since she suffers from untreated scoliosis, she's bent like a candy cane. She can't walk any distance and can't hold or lift anything of any weight because her center of gravity is off. Picture her trying to help a 6'5" man who weighed around 200 pounds, a man who grew more and more frustrated because he forgot how to do things as simple as get out of a recliner.

I don't know if he was impatient with her or if they just lost their balance, but he came down. Fortunately he landed on the couch beside the recliner and wasn't hurt physically. Emotionally and mentally it resembled a mugging. Alzheimer's chose that moment to take one more thing from his mind, and his body paid the price. He was as helpless as he was when he was one year old in 1920.

He seemed to be contemplating everything that had happened that afternoon, but maybe he was grieving. Grieving happens over loss, and he stayed in a constant state of loss. I tried to imagine grieving with no relief. It would finish me.

He began to lose us as his family. About this time, Mama sent several emails that said Dad had asked who she was, or he'd said things like, "thank you, whoever you are." They had been married 58 years. He began to forget who his children were, too. If he didn't know who we were, did our adoration and visits and care speak love to him?

In any visit with Daddy, the conversation turned to WWII. One day when I and the girls stopped by, he talked about three separate war incidents, but they became one story all blended together. War images wouldn't leave, but everything good and worthwhile marched right out of his mind. It was ironic that what he remembered was a war, when there he was, engaged in the greatest battle of his life while Alzheimer's stole the ammunition. It was 1945 and there had been a coup against my dad.

Confusion was the norm now. One morning Martha went to see Mama and Daddy. She walked in on them while Daddy asked the blessing for their breakfast. Everything sounded fairly normal, which was a blessing in itself since he had begun to stumble more with his words. However, he'd prayed for many years and talking with God was not unfamiliar to him. Normal turned to confused though, which is what Alzheimer's does. He closed his prayer and said thank you for a particular mercy, then said "bye bye." God knew.

Fourteen days later, Mom looked for Daddy to brush his teeth and found him on the phone in the kitchen. He was hard to see at first because he stood in the doorway between the kitchen and the living room. Mom said, "Oh, did somebody call?" He said, "Yes." "Who is it?" Mom asked. Dad hesitated. "No . . . I'm trying to call . . ." She was curious and prompted him. "Who?" He said, "I'll . . . show you." Then he pointed to the overhead light at the end of the living room. Mom finally figured out what he was doing. "You're trying to turn the light on?" To which he responded, "Yes."

Alzheimer's was such a demeaning way to die.

My Heritage

Two weeks later, in the middle of November, Dad got in an argument with the recycle men because they didn't also pick up the garbage. Later when he heard the trash truck coming he said he was going out to see about it. Mom told him to wait and leave them alone but he wasn't interested in waiting. Her request held him up long enough that the garbage men had emptied the garbage and started down the road before he got to the end of the driveway.

He didn't know Mom watched the whole thing from a window. When he returned to the house, he said, "Well, I got them straight" (in his best sergeant's tone). He hadn't said a word to them. Mom was gracious and just quietly told him she was glad. Sternly, he said, "I am too!"

Was there a right way to deal with this kind of situation? Garbage men meet all kinds of people, and I'm sure they wouldn't have hurt him. We hated that it looked like he was picking a fight, but we couldn't have changed anything short of putting up a banner that said "A man with Alzheimer's lives here" and hoped they understood.

It had been just one year since Dad wrote the anniversary card for their 57th anniversary, the rose among thorns, but somehow it was sixty-one years earlier, before Dad met mom. The real date was November 25, 2003. It was any body's guess when he thought it was. On that day, I was impressed to go by their house before work. I debated on not going, or going at 3:00, even tried to convince myself I might go after work. I decided to just go and not let anything get in the way.

I called from the drive way so I didn't startle them. When I got in the house I thought it smelled like poop, but didn't think anything of it. I noticed their bedroom door was closed so I waited in the hall. I even made use of the bathroom so they wouldn't find me just standing outside their bedroom door. When I came out and went into their bedroom, Daddy was sitting in his underwear. That's all. I joked to him, "I hope you're going to put on more clothes than that because it is *cold* outside!" We all laughed.

He started trying to tell me about something awful he had done. He'd had diarrhea in the bed and hadn't even realized it. They found it when he got up this morning. The bed was a mess. He'd already had his shower and was waiting to get dressed. I told Mama I would strip the bed for her. While I was doing that, she asked Daddy to get up on the bed so she could rub the cream on his legs. He'd had circulation problems in his legs since before I was a little child. Forty or more years of circulation problems caused the skin to break down, become inflamed, and itch. He would claw them which made them worse. Thankfully the cream helped but it was very difficult for Mom to apply it because of her scoliosis.

While Mom rubbed the cream on his legs, he started crying. Crying so softly and saying in broken sentences that he had done something terrible, how awful it was. Almost in the same breath, he said, "Thank You Lord for these ladies who care for me. Thank you for their kindness." Crying. Mama and I tried to comfort him. I told him he had two surprises that day. One was bad (the messed up bed) and the other was good (my coming by).

It went on and on like that. He stopped for a while. I worked on getting him dressed, and while he buttoned his shirt, I started the mattress cover, treated the sheets, and got the jeans drying again because they were still damp. When I came back, we started on his socks. Those socks were a workout! I don't know how Mama ever managed them with her back bent like it is. At one point Dad started crying again. Then Mama cried with him. His was soft, hers were more like sobs. It broke my heart.

She had mentioned that today was their anniversary. Fifty-eight years. When I mentioned it to Dad, he didn't even know who he was married to. When I told him he was married to Mama, he started crying again. "Thank you Lord for these kind ladies who care for me," he said. That's when Mama started sobbing. "Thank you Lord for sending these people," he said. Mama said, "And I didn't even ask for help. What do you know, honey . . . yesterday, we read the verse that said, 'Before you call, I will answer.'" [3]

This was my heritage. These two people, my parents. Such a mercy of God to me.

I wish I could have done more to ease the hardness of their lives. They expended all their energy just to make it through the basics like dressing, eating meals, taking medicine, being clean, and going to bed. Every moment was about survival *because life was more precious than anything*. Every evening they were physically, emotionally, and spiritually spent. Every morning, they fought for life all over again.

---

[3] Isaiah 65:24.

December Decline

January 2nd had been the best day of the year. December 1st was the second best day of the year. Between those two dates, we had tumbled down the hill of decline just as fast and messy as you can imagine getting in wet South Carolina red clay. For one brief moment on this second best day of the year, Dad was lucid and carried on this conversation with Mom.

Mom was in the kitchen cleaning up when Daddy came in. He said, "Honey, when . . . uh . . . did you first notice that . . . something was wrong with my memory?" She was dumbfounded because they hadn't been discussing his health at all. So many times before he had said things like, "I don't understand why I can't remember" this or that. Mom told him the first time she knew there was more wrong than just old age forgetfulness was when Nell's daughter had died. That was before August of 1998. He thought on that and said, "It's been a slow, gradual thing then." This was the most intelligent, in depth conversation Mom and Dad had had in months, maybe since January second or before.

He was sensible for the most part for at least a couple of hours more. It made our hearts light for a moment, Mom's especially. When she told the family in an email, this was her testimony: "I don't know how long it will last but I just wanted you all to know it and rejoice with me for now."

One person was called to die a hard death and the other was called to live a hard life. They both chose grace for their calling.

Later that same day, Daddy talked to Mom again and said, "You know, Warren's lost interest in me. That must be why . . ." his voice trailed off but picked right back up. "He used to take me to church . . . spend time with me . . . did things with me . . . and he doesn't any more. That must be why." He repeated the last sentence to convince himself. Mom explained to him that Kaaren had been taking them to church because it was too hard for Mom to get them both ready in time for Sunday school. Warren's family had faced a number of health issues that fall, and Warren ran his own business. It was not a loss of interest that kept him away. Dad cried and said he appreciated Mom explaining these things to him. Mom was glad he had brought it up so she could put his fears to rest, even if only for a moment. The paranoia of Alzheimer's was crippling.

Eight days before Christmas, December 17th, Mom and Dad were going about their business in the house while men on the roof cleaned the gutters. While Mom cooked breakfast, Dad asked, "What's your name?" Mom replied, "Pat." Dad immediately started crying a little. After a minute, he said, "That makes me cry because that was my mama's name." (Her name was Alice.) And then he sobbed.

He remained with Mom in the kitchen but his mind wandered between the past and the present. They ate their breakfast. At some point, he was aware of the men on the roof and was determined to go outside and talk to them. Mom stalled him by explaining June had sent them. He said, "But I want to tell them about my sister that sent them here."

Later that same morning, Dad shaved and then asked Mom to feel his face. He wanted to know if he had shaved well enough for church. Mom explained for the fourth time that that day was Wednesday and not Sunday. They weren't going to church. His body stayed with her but not his mind. A few minutes later, he asked Mom if "this" (pointing to his jeans) was good enough to wear to church. His eyes were as blank as his mind. Shortly after that he wanted to call Warren. Mom asked, "What do you need, honey?" He responded, "I want to see . . . uh-h-h . . . see . . . if we . . . uh-h-h . . . can ride to church . . . with him."

A Habakkuk Kind of Christmas

The declining days of December easily took the Merry out of the Christmas season. They made me think about what it was like to receive a big bag of sorrow as your gift (it would be a really big bag of coal in the vernacular). Habakkuk 3:17 and 18 came to mind. "Though the fig tree should not blossom, nor fruit be on the vines, the produce of the olive fail and the fields yield no food, the flock be cut off from the fold and there be no herd in the stalls, yet I will rejoice in the Lord; I will take joy in the God of my salvation."

I read it like this in my mind: "Although my husband has Alzheimer's, and he stays constantly confused; although he grows more incapable with each passing day and requires constant supervision; although he doesn't know my name even though we've been married for 58 years: will I rejoice in the Lord? Will I joy in the God of my salvation?" A "yes" response to those questions was a real test of faith.

For Christmas, Kaaren and I had decided we'd do stockings for Mama and Daddy. Stockings for our parents were a tradition started back in 1969 by Kaaren's then soon-to-be husband. He was spending Christmas with us and was learning what our traditions were. As kids, we always received stockings on Christmas morning. He turned that tradition right back on us and asked if we had thought about doing stockings for our parents! All of the kids participated and a new tradition was born. Lynn died suddenly in 2001, but we had not forgotten what he started. Money was tight, but we couldn't bear to let go of a tradition that was thirty years old. It was hard enough watching Alzheimer's take everything from Daddy without losing some of our traditions to it, too. The only reason not to do the stockings was Daddy's health, and the only reason to do the stockings was . . . Daddy's health. Alzheimer's was complicated.

The question was what do you put in someone's stocking who grows more and more confused every day? We talked for a few minutes, and Kaaren thought of putting a few car-related items in there in hopes that it would be something he recognized. I thought of a tire gauge. She thought of WD40. He had used WD40 for all kinds of things in the past, and he was faithful with a tire gauge.

Later Mom described how pitiful it was. When they opened their stockings, Dad was so confused he didn't know how to open the presents, didn't understand what the gifts were, etc. It was sad. Had we actually contributed to pointing out his decline by keeping the tradition alive? Who knows? Did it matter?

Sadly enough, he didn't recognize the things we hoped would bring him the greatest comfort. Just nine days later when Kaaren was helping Mom and Dad get dressed for morning church, she sent Daddy to the bathroom to take care of business. He was gone for such a long time that she decided she should check on him. She found him in the bathroom fixing his hair with the WD40.

Rather than bring comfort, tradition almost brought disaster. It was a Habakkuk kind of Christmas.

Brrr!

Just two days before 2003 was gone, Dad's mind was going with it. Outside was a chilly thirty-seven degrees. Sometime after breakfast, Dad came to Mom with his sweater half off and said, "Brrrr. It's cold." Mom told him, "If you're cold, you ought to put your sweater back on, not take it off." "That's what I'll do," Dad said, and he put the sweater back on. A few minutes later, he took it completely off. Mom told him he must not be cold after all since he took his sweater off. He seemed not to notice. Minutes later, he had taken off his shoes and was running around in his socks. When Mom mentioned this to him, he seemed surprised that his shoes were off and said, "I guess I'll . . . uh-h-h . . . put them back on." He didn't. Not long after this conversation, Mom found him with one leg out of his jeans. She said something to him, but he was confused about everything. He put the jeans back on and Mom gave him his shoes. He put the shoes back on. She asked him if he wanted his sweater, but he decided he wasn't cold. (Dad was always cold.)

His confusion and disorientation all seemed to start with his comment about how cold it was. A sweater is what you wear when your mom is cold. Dad's mom wasn't there to decide for us and we could have used her! It was so hard to make a decision for a non-functioning adult. In the end, he didn't catch pneumonia running around with no sweater, but his discomfort was our discomfort. His burden our burden. His sorrow and sadness, our own. Goodbye to some hard days. Hello to some harder days in 2004.

2004 — Further Retreat

115 Hale Drive

Happy New Year.

On January 4th, Mom was startled awake by Dad at 5:00 a.m. up on one arm. He barked in his most commanding sergeant's voice, "Sir! Who are you?!" When no answer came and he realized Mom was awake he said, "Somebody called us at that window [their side window]. Somebody's there." Mom calmly said, "Oh, I don't think so."

Instantly she realized she shouldn't have said that. She wished she had said something like "Well, you scared them off" but she hadn't. Dad flopped down on the bed. "Mama . . . I knew you wouldn't believe me." His heart pounded and he breathed hard for fifteen or twenty minutes. Eventually he went back to sleep. Thankfully, there wasn't anyone calling Mom and Dad through the side window. Logically, if someone wanted to get their attention, they would come to the sliding door, and if someone meant harm or were being sneaky, they wouldn't call out. Nothing was logical to Daddy at this point in time nor could he separate between reality and imagination. He couldn't reason anymore, but once upon a time, no one reasoned better than he did.

2004 started off in fine Alzheimer's fashion.

January 10th was like most days in an Alzheimer's year, as ridiculous or weird as *Alice in Wonderland*. Kaaren was busy with a hunt club breakfast, so I volunteered to take Mama grocery shopping. Kenny went with me to Daddy-sit. Dad couldn't be left alone for even a minute. Maybe we were too cautious, but it only took a few minutes for something to happen.

I picked up Wendy's for lunch because it was cheap and Mama and Daddy liked Wendy's nuggets and baked potatoes. Mama fixed some beets so they could have their dinner at lunch time. Daddy seemed to be fading from us at an alarming rate. Actually, *we* seem to be fading from *him* at an alarming rate. Us, normal daily activities, life in the ordinary every day sense of the word were all walking right out of his mind without even so much as a backwards glance, it seemed.

We sat down to eat our Wendy's dinner. We fixed his salad, potato, biscuit, hot tea, and cold Coke. All of it. We put his fork under some food so that when he lifted it up, if he was steady enough, he'd end up with a bite. Sometimes we told him what was on his plate. "This is potatoes, Daddy. Yummy potatoes with butter and sour cream." Or, "I've cut up some ham for you, Daddy. Sherry brought ham today, and it's wonderful. Right here's a biscuit to go with your ham, and some potatoes and cheese." The fancy name of hash brown potato casserole was too much to take in. He forgot all of it. The sweet and sour sauce for dipping nuggets in, he tried to pour on his potatoes. He was just as apt to stab a biscuit with a fork as he was to pick up boiled potatoes with his fingers. None of it made any sense to him anymore.

None of it made any sense to me either.

After dinner, Mom and I shopped while Kenny stayed with Daddy. Kenny likes to be busy, so I'm sure he had a hard time sitting and listening to stories, reading to Daddy, or watching the *Sound of Music*. Later, Kenny told me he got the grandfather's clock running again. He also made their bed for them and filled up the bird feeder.

When we got home with the groceries, Daddy helped me unload the car. I noticed his beautiful Swiss government watch was a third of the way up his arm over his sleeve. It looked like he had showed it to Kenny and, while trying to straighten out the band, had worked it higher and higher up his arm. We finished unloading the car.

Hours later Mama called. It was past their bedtime, about 8:45, and she was upset. She couldn't find Daddy's watch anywhere. I was thankful that I had noticed his watch on his arm. I asked some simple questions: did you go out after I left? Has any trash been taken out since I left? Have you washed any clothes? No, no, and no, she said. Tears and her voice rose a little. She was upset because she couldn't find that watch. More tears. It had been a hard day.

She had told me this morning when they were getting dressed that Daddy asked her what her name was. She said "Pat." He said, "That's so exciting. My wife's name was Pat." Two strangers lived in that house. Mom was a stranger to Dad, and he to her. I don't remember where the watch was found. It became inconsequential in light of losing some of Daddy every day.

A man with Alzheimer's lived at 115 Hale Drive. Not the man who loved people, who was strong enough to be gentle, was as consistent as the tides, and adored his wife. He visited every once in a while, but if we weren't paying attention, we missed him.

A Familiar Stranger

Mom and Dad had been married fifty-eight years, but Dad didn't know Mom anymore. She had become a familiar stranger to him. When they were alone, he could be resentful and ugly with her. My dad was the godliest man I know, but a partial picture of Alzheimer's would be misleading. Dad had a kind heart. He wasn't a pushover or a pansy, but he had a kind heart. Rudeness was foreign to him and he was Webster's definition of a gentleman.

The morning of January 15th was a different story. It was the definition of an Alzheimer's day in all its ugliness. Dad had a dermatologist's appointment at 10:15. At breakfast, he was determined he wasn't going to drink his water for his medicine. Two different pills each required a full glass of water. Mom was willing to let him do one glass for both pills. That morning he was more obstinate than usual, even pouring some of the water out on the table. Mom stopped him. He stood up and was *not* going to drink it. He finally sat down after a long time, but took tiny little sips at long intervals. They were barely ready to go when June got there for the dermatologist's appointment.

One of their granddaughters moved in with them about the middle of January. We hoped a new "stranger" in the house would help the dark, ugly days diminish.

The Dressing Routine

Close to the end of January, I was able to spend part of four different days with Mama and Daddy. Sunday dinner had originally been planned for a relative's visit, which didn't happen. We had the dinner anyway: my ham that was already bought and Kaaren cooked broccoli and cheese. Monday, I was off work for Martin Luther King Day and had volunteered to take Mama and Daddy to the dentist for cleanings. Thursday I came by to help Daddy get dressed and give Mom some relief. Saturday, Kaaren had to work so I took Mama grocery shopping.

I don't remember a whole lot about Sunday. Daddy had been sick the night before. We limited his vegetables and his dessert at Sunday dinner so we didn't contribute to a sensitive system. Limiting the vegetables was no problem; the dessert was another story. He wasn't ugly but he wasn't happy over that decision, either. Maybe because we were there, he didn't react rudely to Mama.

Three of the days, I ate with one or both of them. Meal time was medicine time. Daddy put up more and more of a fight about taking his medicine. I don't think he missed any dosage, but some of the incidents were plain ugly. Mama said one time she tried to get him to take his medicine, but he was obtuse about the whole thing, and poured his water on the table. My dad! He *never* would have done anything like that before Alzheimer's took up residence.

That was the naked truth about the disease. It robbed. We were so conditioned to think of robberies as something to guard against from the outside. This robber was inside, which meant we were unprepared. We couldn't see it happening until the robbery had already occurred. We were left with what the thief didn't want. Isn't that how robberies always are?

49

The more Dad was robbed, the more precious what was left behind became. On many occasions Mama said that he called her "that lady." I noticed on Thursday when I was over there in the morning helping him get dressed that he called me "that lady." About half the time, he didn't know who I was. That was okay. I knew who he was, and he couldn't help it. Sometimes he asked me how many children I had. If I was over there for lunch, he'd ask if my kids needed to eat. He'd also ask if they had to go to school and what their names were.

Monday of that week, I went over there to help them get ready for the dentist, take them to the appointment, and then spend as much time as I could with them until the kids were out of school. I drove my car because I wanted to run errands but my car was small for Dad. He got a cramp in his thigh trying to pull his long legs into the backseat. He was always so gracious about any discomfort, and this time was no exception. I got the seatbelt on him. He didn't know how to do that anymore, and hadn't for a long time. He also didn't know how to work a car door. They all opened differently, and nothing looked familiar or made any sense.

Once we arrived at the dentist, Mama told the receptionist that they were there for their cleanings. Daddy shuffled to the chairs and I got him to sit down. Before long, a hygienist took them back. She told me to come back by 12:30. They would be done by then. I noted the time and got on my way.

Daddy was done first and his hygienist brought him just outside the lobby. I met them in the hall and took Dad's arm so he would follow me to the chairs in the waiting room. After we sat down, he heard Mama's voice. "Who's she talking to?" he asked. I said it must be the lady cleaning her teeth. Then he heard Dr. Healey's voice. "Is that the doctor?" he wanted to know again. I said yes. He had just seen Dr. Healey about three minutes before. Mama's voice. Dr. Healey's voice. Mama's voice some more. I could see Daddy thinking. I mentioned that Mama was talking to the doctor.

Daddy said, "She must have a lot more to say than I do." Then he looked at me very knowingly, but not a nice knowingly, and said, "I don't know when she'll stop. I guess when there's not anything else left to say, because she has a *lot* to say" and nodded his head at the end while he commented. I knew he meant all the things she said to him from time to time. It broke my heart how he viewed her. They were a team, looking out for the best interest of each other. Now she was in the way of everything he wanted to do. We knew she was trying to take care of him. He thought she was trying to control him, and couldn't understand that control was care in this case. It was just spelled differently.

I told him, "She's trying to negotiate a deal with the dentist because it's a new year. She's asking him about medical insurance she saw that includes dental insurance . . . wondering if it's a good idea." Her job wasn't easy, for sure. I tried to put as positive a spin on the situation as I could.

Finally we finished at the dentist and headed home for lunch. Daddy prayed over the meal like he always did. I'd noticed a huge difference in his prayers over the last six months. They were uncertain. They were faltering. Sometimes they didn't include the food. Thank God that "the Spirit knows how to make intercession for us" [4] whether it's physical limitations or spiritual limitations. My dad was always a man of prayer. At this point in time, he still prayed every day with Mom, but often he apologized to God for his behavior or even for imagined things. "He knows our frame. He remembers that we are dust." [5]

Thursday morning I showed up unexpectedly to help Daddy get dressed. He was still in the shower, but I could tell Mama was glad I was there. Thankfully, she seemed fairly chipper and Dad seemed glad to see me when he got out of the shower and dried off. I did a mental exercise to see if I could remember his dressing sequence. I forgot the first and most important thing: his nitroglycerin patch. I did remember to have his t-shirt on the heater warming up. Mom was impressed by that. On it all went. The patch, the warm t-shirt, the cream on the back of his legs, socks, long johns, shirt, pants, and finally the shoes. I had to help him buckle the belt, and a couple of times he tried to put the wrong shoe on his foot, but we straightened that out. Finally, I took him into the bathroom to comb his hair, and we were done.

This was the first of many days to come. Me and Dad and the dressing routine.

---

[4]   Romans 8:26.
[5]   Psalm 103:14.

Humbled by a Kleenex

O ne Saturday at the end of January, we scheduled Dad for a haircut in order for Mom to grocery shop. Warren handled the haircut appointment and I handled Mom and the grocery store.

There was no way Mom could get Dad dressed for his appointment and get herself ready in time to leave at 7:15 for the grocery store. She asked me to be at their house by 6:45. I gulped. I lived twenty-five minutes away which meant I'd have to leave my house at 6:20 a.m. However, I only had to do that once, while the hardship my parents lived with happened every day.

They were still asleep when I arrived. They got up in such a hurry, I was afraid that one or both of them would get hurt. Warren wouldn't fuss at Dad if he was running behind a few minutes, I felt sure. Mama asked me to get the hot water going in the bathroom, and then she took over with Dad who was stripped down to his underwear and socks.

I heard Mama's voice rise with panic from where I was on the outside of the bathroom door. Dad was about to get in the shower with his underwear on. If she tried to stop him, I could see them both going down on the floor. Disaster was averted, but only for a moment. Once the underwear was off, I heard panic again. The socks were about to get a bath. My bent mom tried to stop the Alzheimer's madness and somehow succeeded. I was still on the other side of the door, so I didn't witness how they both stayed upright. Mercy was the only possible answer.

That morning I put his nitroglycerin patch on him for the first time. I had it out of the box and the package ripped open. I also had his t-shirt draped over the electric radiator heater to warm it up for him. When he finished showering, Mama dried off just the bare necessities to get him decent in clean underwear. When they finally came out of the bathroom, she handed me the towel and asked me to finish drying him off.

I tried to imagine what it would be like to have fought in five battles, seen atrocities like the Jewish death camps, watched soldiers from your own unit get blown apart, and suddenly not be able to manage a towel. Also, most people like to dry off a certain way. I didn't know how he liked to dry off. It wasn't something we talked about when his mind was clear.

We dried his chest, back, underarms, and legs all the way down to his ankles. Once that was done, the nitroglycerin patch was next. I became frustrated because I couldn't get the back off. He stood there cold and patient while I figured it out. Finally the patch cooperated but I could see the faintest fingerprint on its underside after it was on Dad. I made a mental note to myself not to use lotion before handling the patch next time. Would the oil from the lotion affect it? I didn't know, but I wasn't about to rip it off and waste it.

The t-shirt was good and warm by this time. Off the heater it came and on to Daddy. He liked that. I had learned something since a previous time dressing him. He liked to put his arms in first and then pull shirts over his head. Last time we put the t-shirt on I made the mistake of treating him like a child. I put the shirt on his head and then pulled. I said boop! when I pulled it down around his neck and then left it for him to get his arms in the sleeves. He couldn't do it. I reminded myself then he needed help like a child but he wasn't a child. *Always, always treat with dignity and respect. Always.* These words became my mission.

This time around, we did better. He held his arms out and I remembered not to use the "boop" method. The t-shirt went on and then we sat down for the cream the doctor had him use on the front and back of his legs. We sat on the side of the bed for this, side by side. Dad cried because I was there to dress him and things had been in such a rush. He mentioned how wonderful "both you ladies are" referring to me and Mom. I got a Kleenex for his nose.

I handed him the Kleenex and reached for more cream at the same time. He was confused about a couple of things, but I only paid attention to his legs and the cream. While I rubbed, Dad lifted his leg in the air. I wanted it to be easy for him so I gently lowered the leg to the floor. We did this a couple of times. The leg would go up and I would lower it. Finally, with his leg raised in the air again, he said, "Now what . . . uh . . . what am I supposed to do with this?" I said, "Just put it on the floor, Daddy." "O-o-on the floor?" "Yes," I said. "Just put it on the floor." "Okay," very quietly.

He bent over and gently placed the unused Kleenex on the floor. My heart broke. His entire conversation had been about the Kleenex while mine had been about his leg. His nose was running because of the tears, the Kleenex was in his hand, but he didn't know to use it. Something in his manner and the way he said "okay" indicated that he didn't think it made any sense to place the Kleenex on the floor, but he had learned not to trust himself. When he thought he understood, and when he thought he didn't, he couldn't trust himself. He lived in a war zone and he couldn't trust anybody there.

I wanted to forget the humbling of my father, except that I believe it is the number one Alzheimer's atrocity and must be communicated. Alzheimer's took him prisoner. As if that wasn't enough, the disease humbled and degraded, and took him captive into a world that got smaller and smaller while he lost his memory, his ability, and eventually his life.

A Daughter's Experience

I was frantic to get to work. I knew I'd be late because I had helped Daddy get dressed after running to Wal-Mart for Mom. He was not ready to get up when I arrived at my usual time, so I tried to be useful and make the Wal-Mart trip. When I got back from there, Mom had Dad up and in the shower. We dressed in record time. Mama had poured me some juice so I sat down with Daddy and drank it. That only took maybe two minutes at the most, because I didn't stay. When I got in the car, I felt myself pulled down emotionally, deeper and deeper. I had to call my boss and tell her I'd be late to work.

Before I started helping Dad get dressed, I was rarely late. I had a reputation for being at work by 7:30 a.m. or 8:00 at the latest, this in an office that started at 8:30. Now, the trips to their house were changing my arrival time. I had to tell her I'd be fifteen minutes late to work. I thought about this as I drove like a maniac, cutting in and out of traffic, doing 63 mph down a city boulevard with a mild case of road rage, and then illegally parking so I could get my morning caffeine.

Once I arrived at my office's parking garage, I said to myself, *I can't continue doing this. I can't continue being late to work. I'll have to leave Mom's and Dad's house by 8:05, no later. Absolutely not a minute later. I just can't stand to ask* . . . Then it dawned on me. I didn't want to ask for help. I needed something and I had to ask for help from my boss. I didn't like being needy.

This was where Daddy lived. He didn't necessarily have to ask for help but he needed help all the time. I prayed the Lord would lift their spirits that day in spite of it all. Dependency created such tension.

True Love Day

Valentine's Day usually falls on February 14th. In 2004, it came on the 4th. Such a tender moment. I don't know when I'd seen anything like it. In fact, the morning was full of tender moments. Mama waking Daddy up, their hands touching and ending up in a tender clasp. Mama giving Daddy his pill, and putting her hand on his back to support him while he leaned on one elbow to take his medicine. The sweetest moment, though, was when Daddy and I walked down the hall. He saw Mama walking towards him and they literally walked into a hug, the sweetest I've ever seen. Both of them stooped, her more than him, so that he was towering above her. Her head was barely at his shoulder. The words "tender" and "love" were defined in that moment. Not raging passion. Not romance. But love from Mama that said when you don't think you can go any longer, I'll go with you until I'm spent. When you're helpless, I'll help you until I'm used up. A love from Daddy that said when I don't recognize you, I still recognize your care for me. I'm overwhelmed by it even though I'm uncertain sometimes as to who you are and why you do what you do.

This was the love language of marriage vows lived out.

His and Hers Troubles

They were a little ahead of schedule when I arrived, so there wasn't much to do as far as dressing. I made myself useful, set the table, and got pancakes ready for breakfast. I poured Daddy some juice and had him drink it as I got breakfast ready. While Mama's pancakes warmed up, she read the verse from the box, and then asked Dad to pray. He sat there for a few seconds. He started, but didn't get more than four words out. Since I was in the kitchen, I couldn't hear well above the noise of the microwave. I do know, though, that his voice didn't continue; whether he was crying or didn't know what to say, I couldn't tell. Finally Mom said, "Would you like for me to pray, honey? Okay, I'll pray."

A few days later, I arrived at their house about 7:08 a.m. As I walked toward their bedroom, I could hear Mama's voice and her grunts. When she saw me she was so obviously relieved, that I thought I must be late, or maybe Daddy was hurt or not cooperating. She had been putting the cream on the back of Daddy's legs, which meant she had already done the nitroglycerin patch, the short-sleeved t-shirt, and the long john t-shirt. She said something like, "Oh! there you are! I was wondering if you were coming this morning. Almost started to call you. In fact, had the phone book out, but you're here finally. Thank the Lord for that!"

Finally? It was only eight minutes after 7:00! I finished dressing Dad, and after I saw the condition Mama was in, her comments made more sense. Her arthritis and scoliosis were so bad I don't know how she didn't fall in any of her attempts to help him get his clothes on.

In spite of Alzheimer's, arthritis pain, and weakness, the next day Dad hummed ever so slightly in the shower. Just the barest hum, not intended to be heard. While he dressed, he did it again. The barest audible hum. I'm not even sure what the song was, but it struck me that I didn't know anyone who had a song in his heart as much as my Dad. "Making melody in your heart to the Lord." [6]

---

[6]   Ephesians 5:19.

March Madness

March blew in. One particular day when I was with Daddy, I was saddened to see that Alzheimer's laid siege to common courtesy. Without knowing my dad, the impact of this statement would mean nothing. He was always selfless, and a gentleman's gentleman, especially with the ladies. Mom's hip and back were in a terrible state, some of the worst I'd seen. She tried to give him his medicine and a drink. Just standing beside him was difficult and painful. In spite of her condition, he persisted in making a big deal about drinking the water until I thought she would fall. He wasn't even aware of her pain. I'm not talking about remembering a discussion of her pain just minutes before. No discussion was needed for someone to be able to tell she was in pain. I'm talking about a simple observation of body language, from watching her face drawn up, listening to her breathing more rapidly and shallower, her trembling, etc. None of these signs indicated anything to him about her condition.

Alzheimer's rode in on a mule and sent chivalry packing.

A few days passed. Dad was in much more of a daze than he had been. The worst moment of the day came in the evening when he asked Mom who all those people were on the couch (in the den). Mom was in the kitchen and asked, "Who?" He pointed through their pass-through towards the couch and said, "There." Mom told him she didn't see any people and asked him where they were again. He pointed back at the couch and said, "They're moving all around." He was *sure* they were there.

Dad's hallucinations unnerved Mom. Eventually he said, "Well, forget it," and he seemed to do just that. The mix of hallucinations and paranoia continued during the night, so sleep was interrupted and nerves were frayed.

One March morning Mama told me that during church the last two Sundays, Daddy whistled all the songs in the service. She didn't know whether to stop him or to let him continue. He whistled them perfectly, but people turned around to look at him.

I thought she handled it remarkably. If he had been with me at my church, I would have been uncomfortable and would have tried to stop him, and I felt sure people would have stared.

Friday night of the same week, she called me in tears after they had gone to bed. She had gotten Dad dressed for the night, and they'd gone to bed. Four different times, he had taken his pajamas off and gotten back in bed naked under the covers. She had convinced him three times to get his clothes back on. Finally, the fourth time she called me. I talked to him on the phone. I said, "Daddy, this is Mary. Mama says you've taken your pajamas off. Did you take your pajamas off?" He said, "Y-y-yeah." I said, "Why did you do that? You don't normally sleep with your pajamas off. Can't you hear Mama crying there beside you?" He said, "Y-y-yeah." I said, "Do you want me to hop in my car and come over there and get you dressed again, like I dress you in the mornings? I can do that." He said, "N-n-no. I'll put my clothes back on" in a small, child-like voice. I told him, "Put your clothes back on. I guess I'm curious why you did that?" He said, in a very disgusted tone of voice, "Well, there's a u-h-h-h lot of competition here . . . with all these men and these gals." I said, "Well, I'm getting in my car and driving over there. I'll see you shortly. Now, give the phone back to Mama."

I told her I was on my way. She called me after about eight minutes and said, "Daddy's put his clothes on." I said, "I'm going to keep driving and I have to buy gas. That will give you time to decide if things have settled down or not. If you're comfortable that every thing's okay, call me back and I'll go back home. Otherwise, don't be alarmed if you hear the door open."

She called back about ten minutes later. "He's in bed, and seems settled." She was crying, though. I said, "I'm coming anyway."

When I got to the house, I went in and talked to both of them. Mama was crying. Daddy lay beside her rubbing her back. I gave Mama a Kleenex. I went over to Daddy, and said, "You got your pajamas on now? I can't see very well in the dark." He said, "I been bad. I'm sorry . . . caused problems. My clothes are on." I said, "Good!"

Then we talked about the situation a little and why Mama didn't feel like she could call Warren (he'd been sick). I said, "He hasn't been coming over to pray, has he?" She said, "No." I said, "I can do that." So I washed my hands of the gas smell and then came back and prayed for them that God would settle their hearts and minds and give them rest.

As far as I know, God honored my prayer. They seemed to have an uneventful night. Mama had trouble falling asleep until about midnight, probably from being so upset. I told her I'd be over early Saturday morning because I had to pick up Lauren from an all-nighter at the school. I could help Daddy get dressed. She was glad to hear that.

Another week battling Alzheimer's.

Horace and Pat

One morning after breakfast, Dad brought the framed picture of him and Mom taken shortly after they were married. He wanted to know who the lady was with him in the picture. "What is her name?" "Pat." This from Pat herself. Dad said, "Oh. Thank you," and turned to leave. Mom asked him, "Do you know who Pat is?" He looked blank for a few minutes and then said, "Pat . . . Pat . . . it seems like I hear that name now and then. Pat . . . Pat." Then Mom asked him, "What's my name?" He stared at her and then managed, "Are you Pat?" When Mom said yes, he asked, "Are you the lady in this picture?"

Not long after that, as Mom finished an email, he brought the same picture back to her and wanted to know who the people were. Mom said, "He's Horace and she's Pat." He wanted to know who Horace and Pat were so she told him the two people in the picture were Horace Lennon and Pat Lennon. Dad wondered if they were still living. "Yes, they are," Mom said. Then Dad asked, "Where are they?" Mom patted him and said, "There you are." He said, "I'm Horace?" Then he asked her if "that lady" was still living. When Mom told him again that "that lady" was her and that she was his wife, they hugged and Dad cried. Even in the middle of his constant confusion, he managed a "Thank you for clearing that up."

Horace and Pat. I loved the sound of that. I wish I had thought to take a current picture similar to the one he kept carrying around and had given it to him. The picture wouldn't have changed anything for Dad, but I would have felt like I had done something to fight against the disease and bring some small comfort to him.

No Match for Grace

The morning didn't start off very well. Mom and Dad sat down for breakfast, which included morning pills. Mom handed Dad one of his pills along with his cup of water, and Dad did an un-Dad thing. He spit his pill into his water. Mom fished it out and put it back on his spoon but war had been declared. Dad glared at her, not very happy that she persisted with the medicine. After finishing his cereal, he pushed away from the table as if to get up. "Don't you want your toast, honey?" Mom kept things as routine as possible. "Y-y-yes," spoken tersely. He stayed sitting at the table but too far from the table to eat without dropping food on the floor. Mom told him he needed to pull in closer. Dad stared blankly at her. "Pull into the table, honey, so you don't drop your food."

Alzheimer's took over at that moment. Dad grabbed the table and jerked it apart (it had a place to add a leaf for larger crowds). In the few seconds it took him to do that, his face said, "So there!" Mom got out of her seat with some difficulty and put the table back together. When she asked him to pull in closer, he jerked the table apart again. Mom tried to hold the table together and encourage him to pull in, but kindness and thoughtfulness had left a long time ago. Dad's reflexes were instant and he grabbed her arm, inflicting pain. When she tried to push his chair in, he planted his feet on the floor and got angry. She couldn't have moved him anyway because of her scoliosis and his size.

Frazzled nerves, hurt arm, and a hurt heart almost encouraged her to slap Dad but instead she prayed. The phone was close by, so Mom dialed Warren's number. While she was waiting for someone to answer, Dad calmed down. He knew she was using the phone. Finally, he attempted to inch closer to the table and Mom helped him. He ate most of his toast. Although he complied with her request, he was not congenial. Sad tension hung in the air.

When he finished his last bite of toast, Mom gave him the pill that needed to be taken after his meal. His water was gone, and Dad said, "I'll go get . . . some water." She told him, "I can't trust you. Friday, you spit the pill out in the sink and I found it later."

Within minutes of this Alzheimer's display, June came by the house for a moment. Dad went outside for a few minutes with her when she left. As her car was pulling away, he came inside the house and hugged Mom. Contritely, he said, "I love . . . y-y-you. Please forgive me for being so or . . . ornery. I don't know why I . . . was . . . that way. The devil just got into . . . m-m-me. Please forgive me." Of course Mom did. Later she sent June an email and wondered if June had said something to him outside, but she knew June wasn't present at breakfast, so how could she know what had happened?

June told her when she was leaving, Dad followed her and asked, "C-c-can . . . I leave with . . . you?" June knew something had happened. Her response: "Dad, you would be bored watching me do tax returns." Then Dad said he hadn't treated Mom right. "Just do your best, Dad, and take it a minute at a time. Don't think about the whole day, just the minute that you're in. Every minute, go tell her you love her. Go in there right now and tell her that you love her." Dad responded, "She . . . she'll . . . say I'm lying." June said, "Dad, don't talk that way. That's just the devil talking." He cried and turned to leave for the house. June touched his arm. "Now, what are you going to do, Dad?" "Tell Mom . . . tell her I love her." His posture didn't match his words, though. He was obviously sad and depressed. June didn't remember what she said to him next, but God perked him right up with it. Dad smiled a big smile and marched back into the house.

Grace triumphed over Alzheimer's when Dad remembered to ask Mom's forgiveness and tell her he loved her. It wasn't always that way in the days ahead, but this particular morning ended much better than it started.

Faith Fight

Footsteps shuffled down the hall towards the bedroom where Mom was. Dad's frame came through the doorway with his Bible in his hand. He sat down beside Mom on the bed but didn't say a word. Mom tried to think for both of them and said, "Would you like me to read you something from the Bible?" "No-o-o." Tears. Finally, Dad said, "When . . . we . . . were . . . in . . . t-t-t-the other room . . . with our Bibles . . ." The right words wouldn't come out, and it seemed that what he was trying to say was that he couldn't think of the right words earlier.

Sitting beside her on the bed, Dad said, "I want . . . to . . . confess my sin." Mom was thoughtful for a minute and told him that not knowing the right words wasn't a sin, and it wasn't anything he needed to feel like he had to confess. He was not convinced. "Yes. Yes it is. My heart's just not right." Tears and more tears.

He could not discern the difference between debilitating disease and sin. His "confessions" never gave him any relief. He was more and more aware of his sinfulness but he didn't seem to remember the righteousness of Christ. He just cried more, unable to understand when he did sin that "if we confess our sins, He [God] is faithful and just to forgive us our sins and to cleanse us from all unrighteousness." [7]

Another morning when I was there, Dad cried and said, "I'll never see my daddy again." Tears. I said, "Daddy, one day you'll see him, but you're right . . . you won't ever see him again here. I have a daughter that I won't see again here. In fact, she's with your daddy." We cried together and talked about that for a few

---

[7] I John 1:9.

minutes, and it seemed to comfort him. The next day we talked again about losing those we love. "It's always toughest for the people left behind," I told him. I don't remember when I figured that out. "Whether someone goes away because of war, or goes away because of death, it's toughest on the people left behind." He seemed comforted again, although I realized it was only for a few minutes.

Alzheimer's waged war against our faith and his. Nothing was sacred.

Alzheimer's Happened

D addy seemed so much better than he had in a week. One morning during the dressing routine, I had the socks started on his toes. He said, "That's gooood." I laughed and said, "Those are becoming my favorite words!" All three of us laughed at that. Because the socks were support hose for bad circulation, they were tighter than a drum and required a fair amount of effort to get them up his legs. While I was tugging and pulling, Daddy said, "I'm at your mercy. You're so gracious." I said, "Yes, Daddy, you spend a lot of time at other people's mercy, and being at someone else's mercy is not very easy. It can be hard." Mama agreed.

All of it brought tears to my eyes. For all my efforts to capture him and his last battle, it wouldn't be enough. Even if I had followed him around and wrote without interruption, I couldn't have captured the sadness of it all or the steps downward into total separation. That's what happened. He forgot everything and eventually become separated from all that was dear.

On Wednesday, Dad asked me who my daddy was. I reached up and patted his knee and said, "You're my daddy." He said, "Really? Really?" His incredulity and seeming happiness touched me. Then he cried. I tried to imagine not knowing my Daddy. I spent quite some time in that frame of mind when I realized I had it wrong. What if I couldn't remember my *children*? My Kenny, or my Lauren, or my Abby. They bring such pleasure to me just through their lives. I couldn't imagine losing *all* the people I loved.

Some days later, this scene greeted me. Dad was convinced he had hurt Mom and kept apologizing and crying. She was crying, too. She told him, "You haven't done anything wrong" over and over. He apologized more. Cried more. Talked about his daddy some more and cried some more. We were all crying at some point. Mom got him in the shower and Daddy almost walked out of the bathroom naked. I hadn't taken over his shower routine yet, so Mama got up as quickly as she could. I watched her face and saw her shake her head. Her mouth moved to tell me something but her mind made her head to the bathroom and pull the door behind her.

In the bathroom, I heard bits and pieces. Daddy: "Was last night a uh . . . dream . . . or uh . . . did that really happen?" Mama: "It wasn't a dream. It really happened." Daddy: "I'm so sorry. We had a time, didn't we?" Mama: "Yes, we had a time." Daddy: "We had a time . . . I'm sorry I did that . . . to . . . you." My heart quickened. This statement conjured up images in my mind that were vague, fortunately, because I've never witnessed my dad being violent to my mom. Daddy timidly came into the bedroom for me to put his patch on him and Mama took her turn in the shower.

Before any water came on, the tears were flowing inside and outside the bathroom. Daddy's head and voice lowered. "We had a time. I can't believe . . ." his voice trailed off and then came back, "what I did to her. It was a time. I'm so sorry. I don't know if she'll . . . ever forgive me." I listened to this for a few minutes. When he kept repeating the phrase "what I did to her," I put my hands on his arms and looked him in the face. "Daddy, you didn't hurt Mama, did you?" I asked him point blank. He looked me square in the face, and said, "Oh no! No . . . I . . . uh . . . didn't. Well, I'm sure I hurt her-r-r . . . uh . . ." he fumbled for the word. I offered up, "Hurt her heart?" He finished with, ". . . hurt her feelings, but I-I-I didn't hurt her."

We had the patch and t-shirt on at this point. Uncertainty and anxiety hung in the air. I didn't know what had happened. Daddy didn't know what to do next. I patted the bed and he sat down. I rubbed the cream on, my hands moving in gentle circular motions so I didn't hurt his tender skin, my mind racing in wild circular patterns with thoughts like *what did he do? what happened? what should I do?!* Mama cried while she undressed and got the water going in the shower. The water flowed from the shower head and the tears flowed from her. Sobbing. A broken-hearted Mama and a broken-hearted Daddy, and a daughter who didn't know what to do.

Daddy was contrite. "I want to ask her to forgive me. I want to do that." I said, "That's the right thing to do. You should do that." I still didn't know what happened. I worried that he'd hurt her somehow, that she'd had to struggle with him even though there were no marks evident. "Should I do it now?" "Now would be good," I said. "Can I go in there?" "Yes, you can, Daddy."

He got up slowly in his underwear, t-shirt and 6th Armored shirt and walked to the bathroom. "Hello, dear. I-I-uh . . . want to ask . . . you uhhm . . . to forgive me. I'm . . . s-s-so sorry. Will you forgive me?"

What I heard next stunned me. Mama said, "Honey, please don't apologize. You've already done it a hundred times before." Sobs made it hard to understand. I'm confused. Done what? Then I realized, he had apologized to her a number of times already and he didn't remember. I didn't find out until later what happened.

What am I saying? Alzheimer's happened.

The sad reality behind the morning's events was Dad dreamed his dad came to see him. At 5:20 a.m. that morning, he got up and took his pajamas off, trying to get dressed so he could go see his dad. Mama was startled awake only to realize Dad wasn't in bed beside her. His absence combined with the darkness terrified her. Where could he be? When she found him, his demeanor was disconcerting. He insisted he wanted to see his daddy and he hummed in a high pitched voice. After being awakened unexpectedly, the terror of not knowing where Dad was, and the sadness of it all, Mom was in tears by the time I got there for the morning routine.

Lunchtime was no better. The car was out of the carport at 115 Hale Drive. I asked Mama if they had been somewhere. They had. Dad wanted to take a walk and promised Mom he wouldn't go past Court Street, a small side street just a block from the house. Mom watched as he walked right past Court Street and kept going. She knew she couldn't run after him so there was nothing else to do but go after him in the car. Dad almost made it to the top of their street which connected to a busy main artery. When she caught up to him, he refused to get in the car, but he did turn around and go back home. She drove behind him all the way back to the house. It is not a long distance, but at two mph and with Dad's unpredictability, it was long enough. When I arrived for lunch, Mama seemed better than she had been that morning but Daddy was still crying.

Medals from the Sixth Battle

D ad was bored and wanted legitimate activity to occupy his time. That prompted an email from Mom:

> *If I thought he'd be fooled with the empty razor I'd let him go to it, plastering on all the shaving cream he wanted but I don't think he'd be fooled. In fact, I think he'd probably open it up and see there was no razor. He's wanting so bad to do something so I gave him three ears of corn to shuck. He couldn't do a single one. He kept saying he wasn't strong enough anymore but that wasn't it. He didn't understand what to do. I showed him and showed him and even started them but he still couldn't do it. He started crying and brought his army picture out of the living room and said, "That's me. Things are different now. I used to be able to do things."*

When I helped Daddy get dressed one morning, June's dog Abby sat on the floor right in the middle of us. Daddy asked me where June was. I was glad he realized Abby belonged to her. I said "Today, she's having lunch with the British Ambassador." He looked at me and said "No kidding? Really?" I said "Yes!" He thought for a minute, his eyes staring straight at the floor. "Well . . . I guess she has to have lunch somewhere!" We both burst out laughing. My dad had visited for a sentence and I was there to see him.

On June 23, 2004, Daddy asked me to tell each one of his children that he sent his love. I told him I would. That day was the 60th anniversary of his watch presentation. He was the saddest I'd seen him in several months . . . crying over the Nazis he killed. Understand, Daddy had killed Nazis when necessary, and believed he was doing his God-given duty fighting for his country. But when the battle was over and the enemy was a prisoner, that wasn't the time for killing.

He talked repeatedly that his lieutenant made him kill a Nazi. "I didn't want to kill them [more than one]," and he cried some more. Later, I asked Ken if he had heard Daddy talk about killing Nazi prisoners that his lieutenant didn't want to take as prisoners. Ken hadn't heard him tell any such story, but he felt sure it was a real possibility. I thought so too. Our speculation was that all these years he'd dealt with it by God's grace, but Alzheimer's revealed what he had kept private. Or maybe his messed up mind confused his memory.

We would never know but it made more sense then why he often told the story about the Nazi soldiers he took as prisoners when he was the one in charge. Remembering that act helped him know when the decision was his to make, he chose life. God helped me think to tell him some duties and responsibilities are easier than others. All are honored by God when we do our duty. The words escaped his mind within seconds, but the dead soldiers did not.

When Daddy handed me what seemed like dirty Kleenex number thirty, he said, "I'm sorry to keep giving you these." All I could think of was that they were a different kind of medal for a battle that was as deadly as any day back in 1945.

You're a Darling

The very next day to those without Alzheimer's was another day at war for Daddy, both in his Alzheimer's battle and in the battle against the Nazi's. 1945 and 2004 were separated by seconds, depending on where his mind was at the time.

Dad rubbed the side of his face thoughtfully. He said to Mama, "Do uh you . . . h-h-have any idea why I . . . have th-th-these little things on my face?"

Mama replied: "Because you're a man. They're whiskers, and all men have whiskers."

Dad (serious and questioning), "They do?"

Mom: "Yep, they sure do."

Dad paused. "I had them when I was . . . over . . . there."

"You sure did, and I bet you didn't always get to shave either."

Dad laughed, lost in time. "No. I sure didn't."

Mom entered his time-frame with him and said, "But you never sent me a picture of you with a beard. All the pictures you sent me you were clean-shaven."

Dad laughed again. "That's right. You're a darling. I th-th-thank the Lord . . . for you!"

And he was right to do so. Not only did she love him by noticing the care he took to shave before a picture, but she cared for and loved his soul. One time he asked me, "Who's the woman . . . uh . . . who's . . . uhhmm . . . so faithful . . . to read the Bible to me?" "Her name is Pat, Daddy." And several times after that, he commented how much he appreciated her reading the Bible to him.

A Book about You

One morning halfway into the summer, while I was helping Daddy get dressed, he asked me again, "Who's your Daddy?" He said it in complete innocence and ignorance, which broke my heart. I was on the floor in front of him helping him get his shoes on. I put my hands on his knees and looked straight at him. "You are. You're my Daddy." I tried to say it with as much emotion and appreciation as I could so he would catch the intensity in my voice.

Immediately his eyes welled up with tears. Quietly, almost as if he dared to hope it was true, "Really? I am?" I got up on the bed next to him and put my arm around him. "Yes," I said. "Yes, you are. And you know what else? I'm writing a book about you!"

He cried. He couldn't believe it. I told him I was writing about what he'd done, what his mother and father did, about our heritage, about God's grace that had been extended to our family, and he sobbed in appreciation. Once he could speak, his first words were, "What . . . what could you possibly . . . write . . . about someone like me?" This was the greatest trait of Daddy's life. True humility.

Hope for Eternity

I'd helped Daddy get dressed in the mornings before work for almost six months now. Most of it was the same. The weather was hotter than when I started, so we were putting on fewer clothes, but we still had to put on t-shirts and shirts, cream the legs, put on socks, pants, and shoes. In the winter, we had to hurry because he was so cold. When I got there on cold mornings, I'd put the t-shirt on the heater to warm it up for him. In the summer? He couldn't understand that no matter how much he dried off, his body stayed damp because of the humidity and the skin's tendency to hold moisture. The entire time we dressed, he dried off.

He seemed more winded with shorter, shallower breaths these days. That concerned me. Sometimes, too, when he was upset (and maybe it was the fact that he didn't feel well or had arthritic pain), he hummed a little hum. Don't think a musical hum. Think "groanings which cannot be uttered." [8] That was what came to my mind when I heard it. The hums were low. They were soft. They were a single tone with a steady rhythm to them.

Groanings which cannot be uttered. When I heard them I thought I knew. I thought I understood. I thought they were the sounds of a broken mind, a hurting body, a crushed spirit. Sounds from within that found their way out.

Since Alzheimer's came into our family, I'd envisioned it as a battle. I thought of it as a lost battle because Dad would die. Nothing except a miracle would stop his death from happening.

The father of one of Ken's friends was put in a home back in late December, early January. Six months passed, and we found

---

8   Romans 8:26 (King James Version), referring to the Holy Spirit.

ourselves in the heat of July. The friend called Ken and said his dad had stopped swallowing and that the family agreed not to allow a feeding tube. Two days later, his dad died. His email shamed me.

"My dad's battle with Alzheimer's is over. He won." [9]

What a beautiful statement of faith in spite of the ugly battle of Alzheimer's. "We have met the enemy and he is us!" [10] Dad fought unknowns because he forgot the known. He fought loved ones because they were strangers. He knew intense fear and uncertainty. He had no way to comfort himself.

Even his soul was not comforted sometimes because he forgot the promises of God. In his mind, he was without God because he couldn't remember he had asked God to save him. Yet God promises absolutely nothing will separate us from His love when we are His.

Through faith in the saving work of Christ, we become dressed in the righteousness of God Himself. "I will greatly rejoice in the Lord; my soul shall exult in my God, for he has clothed me with the garments of salvation; he has covered me with the robe of righteousness . . ." [11] This was Dad's sole hope for heaven, not his own works.

---

[9]   Used by permission from Gary Smith.
[10] Walt Kelly, *Earth Day Poster*, 1970.
[11] Isaiah 61:10a.

Sin, Suffering, and God

Less than a week later, Ken went to Mama's and Daddy's house for what he thought was going to be a few minutes. A few minutes became five hours. When he got there, Daddy was crying. Bawling, according to Ken. Mama was sitting with him but when she saw Ken, she immediately said, "Look here's Ken! Maybe he can cheer you up." Ken said Dad cried for at least twenty more minutes. He couldn't do anything to lift Dad's spirits.

At one point, Daddy talked to Ken about Alzheimer's. He said, "This disease . . . this Altimer's . . . is awful! It's terrible . . . what i-i-t's . . . doing to me. Did . . . I . . . uh . . . do something? Is that why I have Altimer's?"

His question broke my heart when Ken told me. I thought about the blind man in John 9. "And as he [Jesus] passed by, he saw a man blind from birth. And his disciples asked him, 'Rabbi, who sinned, this man or his parents, that he was born blind?' Jesus answered, 'It was not that this man sinned, or his parents, but that the works of God might be displayed in him.'" [12]

I applied it to our present situation: And as the Lord beheld the human race, he saw a man with Alzheimer's. And those who call themselves His disciples asked him, saying, "Lord, who sinned? this man or his parents or maybe his wife, that he has Alzheimer's?" And Jesus answered, "It was not that this man sinned, or his parents, or his wife, but that the works of God might be displayed in him."

"It was not that this man sinned . . . but that the works of God might be displayed in him." Daddy was a confessed believer and follower of the Lord Jesus Christ. He would have no greater

---

[12] John 9:1-3.

joy than for his suffering to be used by God to reveal Himself to . . . you.

Romans says, "For all have sinned and fall short of the glory of God . . ." [13] The wages of sin is death, not suffering in this life. [14] When we think suffering might be payment for sin, we belittle how offensive sin is to God. The cross and the death of Jesus Christ is the reality of sin's offensiveness to God. And yet, ". . . God shows His love for us in that while we were still sinners, Christ died for us." [15] He, who knew no sin, became sin for us that we might be made the righteousness of God! [16] There is *no other way* to God. [17]

---

[13] Romans 3:23.
[14] Romans 6:23.
[15] Romans 5:8.
[16] II Cor. 5:21.
[17] John 14:6.

Alzheimer's Association

Six years into Alzheimer's, we enlisted outside help. The Alzheimer's Association, South Carolina Chapter was a God-send. They were knowledgeable and provided funding for respite care. Everyone in the office had first-hand experience with Alzheimer's and heart-felt sympathy for our situation.

Their first help was to listen as we dumped six years of Alzheimer's pain in their laps in the first phone call. Sherry was the family representative. After her initial contact with them, her email about their empathy and financial aid was like water in a desert. They mailed us a no-expiration-date voucher we could use for sitting fees, etc., so Dad would be cared for and Mom could take a break from being caregiver.

Dad had been growing more and more agitated. They helped us understand this was evidence of another stage of the disease. We were warned that he would become more unsettled and agitated at night. Something about the night created fear and apprehension. Because my time with Dad was almost always mornings, I didn't witness night fears and agitations. Someone did have to deal with them even though they're not recorded in this book, and it was usually my brother Warren, brother-in-law Jerry, or my husband, Ken, and *always* Mom.

The Alzheimer's Association helped us understand that changes in behavior signal a progression in the disease. Shaving could be his favorite activity on Monday, and Tuesday he might not want anything to do with his razor. As he entered the next stage of Alzheimer's, his symptoms might improve for a short time, but then all of a sudden, he would not be able to do something he could do the day before.

They recommended our family attend the support meetings. Some had already attended and found it helpful. Since Mom was the caregiver, it was next to impossible for her to go. AA paid for respite care for her to attend the support meeting. That payment was in addition to the voucher they sent for sitter fees. The Alzheimer's Association was a constant source of help to us. Visit their website for more helpful up-to-date information, www.alz.org.

Perspective

Alzheimer's put things in perspective.

One particular morning, Daddy was different. I wasn't sure what was going on. He was either trying to be covertly hard to get along with or he was completely unable to understand what I said to him. His words were pleasant enough, but it was his attitude. I would say we needed to do something and he would either not do it or mess around and then do it. I mentioned I needed to do his nails because they were long. He went to the bathroom to shave, so I told him I'd get breakfast on the table. I came back in a few minutes to do his nails. Whether he heard me coming or not, I don't know, but I found him trying to shave off his nails. He was running each nail into the head of his razor, back and forth. Did he want to do for himself? Was he tired of being dependent on others? I don't know.

As I made their bed, I thought about recent car troubles and my husband's job loss. My Check Engine light had come on the night before and I was worried about driving the car. Ken had lost his job five months ago. When I remembered Mama in the shower crying, and Daddy shaving his nails, I said to myself, "*Their* problems are problems. My car isn't a problem. Ken's 'no job' isn't a problem. My parents' sufferings are problems."

A Visit to the Doctor

An email from Ken after taking Dad to the doctor . . .

"Good afternoon to the family! We just got back from the follow up visit to see Dr. Kemmerlin. It's rare that you say praise God for a dead battery, but today was such a day. When I went to pull the car out to head to the doctor's office, it wouldn't start. We called Warren and he brought over jumper cables. I was thankful to have his help. We worked for 20 minutes to get Dad in the car. He could not get in and the more Warren and I tried to help, the more he resisted. At one point Dad told us to back off so he could 'kick the door off.' We were able to avoid that. He would lay out across the front seat and push against the door with all his might. On a lighter note, at one point Dad told Warren and me, 'You boys are really confused.' To be honest he about had me convinced!

We finally got him in the car and off we went. When we got to Dr. Kemmerlin's office, Dad was asleep and it was hard to rouse him. I worked for a while and finally got his feet on the ground. At that point he laid back across the seat and started crying and said, 'Why won't somebody help me? Now I'm crying, too, and trying to convince him that I would help him if he'd let me. I was able to get him to stand up. He said, 'I'm going to fall!' I had my arms around him and under his shoulders to support him. He had one of my legs squeezed in between his legs and wasn't going to let go. It was like a bizarre game of Twister. At that point, one of Dr. Kemmerlin's orderlies came out with a wheel chair and we got Dad in the office. This was the most 'resistance' I ever faced with Dad. Based on this and other such situations I think it's a wise decision for a male member of the family to start handling as many of these trips as is humanly possible.

I was glad that Dawn or one of the other ladies was not faced with the situation today. The doctor said everything was doing fine. He talked to Mom about Dad's demeanor and attitude in general. He made two recommendations but other than that he said the status quo was working. Dad got his updated Tetanus shot and the doctor said he didn't have to see him for three or four months unless we needed to. Dad wanted to walk out to the car when we left. He did so and got into the car with little effort. We got home and he is sitting peacefully in the living room listening to some music and whistling right along, completely oblivious to the earlier events of the day. All in all a good doctor's visit and good experience as we prepare to seek some outside help to assist with Dad's care. I'm sending this from Mom's computer so if you want to reply, send it to my home Email not here. I think that about covers the afternoon."

A Merry Heart is a Good Medicine

I stopped by Mom's and Dad's house at lunch one day and was only there about fifteen seconds before I wondered if I had the wrong house. Was this 115 Hale Drive? Mama was laughing, happy, talkative; seemingly untouched by anything that had happened that morning. It was not the same place I'd been going for the last seven months. Her good spirits made all the difference with Daddy. He couldn't do any more, but his demeanor was better.

A big ol' thank you email went to everybody that had contributed to the happiness of the day: Sherry and Jerry, because they got Mama not one but *three* bathing suits for her to try on for her pool exercises; Jerry, for having a birthday and making a good joke on the phone when Mom called so that she laughed; and Kaaren, who pushed Mama to go to the pool when Mom didn't feel like she could. All of them gave her something positive to participate in and enjoy in her hard hours. A shadow was cast over this light mood, though, when I thought about Warren struggling with Dad at night during Dad's sun downing.

One Friday in September, as I helped Daddy get dressed, I mentioned that Kenny had written a speech about him for his freshman speech class. Daddy was surprised and asked what . . . why . . . would he want to do that? Kenny had to pick a hero for a speech topic, and he picked my dad. Of course it made my heart glad. Daddy asked me, "What . . . what's a . . . hero?" God gave me this to tell him. "A hero is a man of great character and courage even in the midst of great fear."

By that definition, my dad was even then a hero.

A few days into October, Dad wanted to shave as usual. We went to the bathroom together and I handed him his razor. When I turned it on and he heard that familiar buzz, he smiled so big and said, "Oh, I love this thiiinnng. Love it! This is my . . . uhh . . . my play pretty!"

Even though his memory was messed up, he was still a connection to the Great Depression and the early 1900's. I was instructed by his thankfulness, appreciation, and enjoyment out of something as utilitarian as a razor. He thought it was a toy, which was probably more of a luxury than a razor was. I never considered myself a historian, but my Dad made me want to know more about the past rather than be so self-absorbed in my own little vapory life span.

October continued with some better days. On the 14th, I got to Mom's and Dad's house earlier than usual. Mama looked like she had already been with her walkin' talkin' ladies at the pool because of her good spirits. Daddy was still having a hard time, definitely going downhill, but he wasn't near as bad as he had been the day before when we had taken him for a flu shot. The change in schedule, rushing around in the early morning hours, must have contributed to his bad morning.

But this particular morning, my son, Kenny, cooked pancakes, bacon, and scrambled eggs while I got Daddy dressed, so breakfast was all ready when we came out of the bedroom. I fed Daddy two whole pancakes with syrup. Kenny's cooking was a distraction to Mom which took her mind off Daddy, which in turn put Dad at ease. Also, Mama had the pool to look forward to, not to mention they were expecting company that afternoon from church. The visitors weren't close personal friends of theirs, but Mama wasn't stressed over it, so that was a blessing. October 14th started out wonderful!

Some of our efforts produced good spirits and some of our efforts were a hard battle just for life to continue the next day. I couldn't thank my brother, sisters, husband, children, and in-laws enough for their shoulders that helped carry Mom's and Dad's burden and sometimes made that burden lighter, if only for a couple of hours at a time.

From High to Low

L ife with Alzheimer's was a roller coaster. Mom was at the end of her rope the early days of December. She stooped with her scoliosis, and her asthma was at its all-time worst, a complication she didn't need. We were on a steep downward slope, so steep it took our breath away.

Just a few days later, we hit bottom (one of many). When I was there, Dad was sure Mom was the enemy. He jumped when she touched him. He begged me over and over "Don't let her get me." I noticed when he was in this state of paranoia, his physical ability left him. He couldn't stand. He'd crawl around the floor. If he managed somehow to get up on his feet, he was unsteady and begged, "Don't let me fall." If he heard something like a closet door closing, he was nervous and asked, "Wh-what's . . . that??? Who's trying to get me?" But, if you could make him laugh, suddenly he could walk, stand up, and was relatively steady on his feet. The effect his demeanor had over his physical condition was hard to believe.

The two days that followed were better. No tears on his part. He was generally cooperative and much more able physically than he had been, although not *real* able. He could stand, though. He wasn't afraid of falling nor was he so disoriented that he couldn't help himself, like use a bathroom counter to hold onto while walking. On his good days, he wasn't able to tie his shoes, and hadn't been able to for about three weeks. On a bad day, he didn't even comprehend shoes or that he needed to do anything with his feet, although he didn't fight me when I tried to put his shoes on him.

When Ken was over at their house during that same week, he sat with Dad on the couch. While they talked, Ken gently rubbed

Dad's shoulder. After a few minutes, Dad turned around and said, "You know what I wish?" Ken said, "What do you wish?" Dad's reply? "I wish you'd stop doing that!"

Alzheimer's at its best.

I'd gone to their house for ten months now. Changes in the weather created monstrous changes in him. They seemed to render him incapable and in pain. Unusual winter weather was forecasted for our area so it hardly seemed a coincidence. One morning, I put his nitro patch on him and walked to the trash can to throw the trash away. He promptly pulled the patch off! He'd never done that before. Once we got another patch on, I walked to the trash can again. When I came back, he had picked up his t-shirt and used it to blow his nose.

These were hard things and we were always unprepared.

Emotions literally bound Daddy or set him free. Mama fell the night of December 16th. No bones were broken, and there were no obvious injuries. She hit her head, but thankfully it wasn't serious. The next day, Daddy was uncertain, shaky, and unsteady on his feet, moaning and saying he hurt. He was an exact reflection of her condition.

When I tried to get clothes on him, he resisted or did things that made it very difficult. He pressed his foot into the floor when I tried to get his long johns on. We put a shirt on that was no good for one reason or another and had to take it off. He held his arms rigid and slightly bent in front of him so it was impossible to take off the shirt. I quit struggling with him and he relaxed, and then I pulled the shirt back up around his shoulders. The resistance could have continued but he quit for some reason. I'd love to say it was skill on my part, but more than likely it was mercy on God's part.

Mama was much better within a few days. She was still in pain but improving. Daddy was much better, too. Congenial. Laughing. Appreciative. *Cooperative.* What a difference. I wondered who got to tell Mom that she couldn't be in pain any more, or depressed, sad, or fearful. No. Too much rested on it.

The downhill progression of the last few weeks got to me Christmas Day. He was so pitiful, left without the means to function. He feared everything.

Help or Hindrance

When I first started going to Mom's and Dad's house, I put Dad's socks on him, his long johns, and pants. He could do those things some days. Did I rob him of some of his abilities because I did those things for him? I considered this after it was too late. He could zip and button his pants, fasten his belt, and tie his shoes when I first dressed him. Now, most of the time, he couldn't tie his shoes. He either tied the shoe strings in a knot or just held them and said, "What do I do with these?"

I'd taken over the bathroom routine by December as well. He couldn't shower by himself and didn't understand what he was supposed to do. Mama fretted about him not getting clean, but he wasn't that dirty. Warren was able to order a case of the rinse-less soap used in hospitals, which was a blessing. If a shower wasn't possible, we used the rinse-less soap. Both shower soap and rinse-less soap dried out his skin, so I tried to remember to put lotion on him. Dry skin itches terribly.

We seemed to move through phases faster. During the summer he went through a phase of doubting his salvation. By December, he forgot to doubt, thankfully. In the summer, he wanted to shave all the time. Within a couple of months, he used the razor like a sander on the bathroom counter. By December, he seemed tired of shaving at times. Other times he went through the motions but held the razor sideways like a sander, sanding his face.

At night, there was so much trouble getting him to bed: fighting, ugliness, a whole different side to what happened in the morning. Sherry and Kaaren both mentioned this. Their mornings were like mine where he was agreeable even though he didn't understand. He rarely fought or resisted a request. Kaaren discovered that speaking softly was the key. I had been talking loudly because he was hard of hearing. I stopped doing that after her discovery, and found if I got close to him and spoke softly, his right ear was good enough that he heard me and he wasn't combative over my requests.

He picked up on hurry and emotions. If I hurried, he became flustered and began to shut down. I couldn't get him to the bathroom, kitchen, car, anywhere! He was strong physically and could hurt every one of us.

He was unable to separate our feelings from his own. Negative emotions incapacitated him physically. His balance was off. He took baby steps or at times crawled. He became unable to communicate, moaning and rocking repetitively. Laughter lifted the physical vise grip of negative emotions, but only for a second.

Eye contact helped communication. He understood more with eye contact, it seemed. Maybe he read facial expressions while he attempted to process words. Whenever I made eye contact with him I saw a spark, if only for a moment.

2005 — Surrender

A Journey Back in Time

"New" doesn't always mean "better." It was a new year, but things weren't better. They were just crazier and sadder and somewhat like time travel. Alzheimer's took Dad back through his life, not a perfect backwards journey in time, but a confused one. Over the course of time, he visited further and further into his past until he was as helpless as a newborn. His end looked strangely identical to his beginning.

Dad's beginning happened in rural eastern North Carolina. He was born to godly parents, Quincy and Alice Lennon, who had seven children over the course of twelve years. Dad was the baby. Quincy was humble, industrious, and ahead of his time. Their home had lights before any other home in that area, and Quincy built the house with a huge closet that he promised would become a bathroom. He knew indoor plumbing wasn't far from reality.

Alice kept the home going in spite of chronic asthma. Not only was she a mother to her own children, but she mothered the motherless, raising grandchildren when one of her own daughters died in childbirth, and opening her home to others who needed a family. Quincy and Alice served their church, cared for their community, and were members of a close-knit family that extended several branches out on the family tree. Part of that close-knit family was Quincy's brother Hardy, his wife, and two of his sons, twin boys named Hubert and Hewlett.

So on January 7, 2005, we somehow found ourselves in the early 1930's.

Everything Daddy did that day, he'd say, "This is Hubert. Now where's Hewlett?" If he was in the bathroom, he pointed to the counter. "Now this is Hubert." Or after he had used the bathroom and then wouldn't let Mama help him get dressed again, he pointed to his depends and said, "Now this is Hubert. Where's Hewlett?" His antagonism to Mom seemed so opposite compared to his concern for and awareness of Hubert and Hewlett. After the bathroom incident, Mom finally gave up and left Dad to make himself presentable again. He came out in the kitchen with his belt undone but other than that he was decent. Mom commented how well he had done. He looked at her, holding the ends of his belt, and asked her to help with "Hewlett."

It didn't stop there. While Mom fixed their weekly medicine boxes, Dad said, "Now that's for the twins, Hubert and Hewlett. Make sure you take care of them."

It was a journey back in time, far away from the present day. It was an old day, a better time.

Battle Cry

"We won't stay here."
Those words comforted when things were bad. In a few instances, loss of memory was a blessing, like no more Germans or incoming fire or anger at your spouse of 59 years.

At other times, those words were a knife in the heart. I'd helped with the morning routine for eleven months. I wanted to turn back the hands of time and go to February of '04, February of 2000, February of '95, but I couldn't. We could only press forward.

"We won't stay here" became a battle cry. When Dad struggled with his salvation, we said, "We won't stay here." When he agonized over Mama's health and became almost catatonic, we said, "We won't stay here." When he could no longer eat, bathe, breathe, we said, "We won't stay here!" Thank God for that. "We won't stay here!" Absent from the body, present with the Lord. [18]

---

[18] II Cor. 5:8.

God's Care

That January morning was hard. Daddy got up before 6:00 to go to the bathroom. He was enough of a mess that he needed his shower then, so he was dressed when I got there. He was either in pain, getting sick, or extremely depressed. In the office, he held my hand and said, "I hope someone . . . I hope everyone . . . cares for you. I hope they do care." We went to the kitchen to get his juice while Mom started her shower.

Walking to the kitchen required effort. He favored his right knee when he got up and when he walked. At the same time, he moaned with a rhythm. Once in the kitchen, he sat with his eyes closed but his face raised to the ceiling. That was not a normal position for him. When his eyes were closed, he usually had his head down as if he were going to sleep. The moaning kept up even after he sat down. Finally he said, "Everyone cares." Pause. "Everyone cares." Another pause. "Except the Lord." It was a knife in my heart. "Daddy, I know it doesn't seem like it sometimes, but the Lord does care. He does care for us." Dad cried at that comment. "Thank you. Thank you. Thank you for that."

Several minutes passed. Whole lifetimes came and went in minutes sometimes so I wasn't sure what was happening in the silence. Quietly I cut up a banana on their cereal. Finally, Daddy said, "No." Pause. "The Lord does care." I was amazed that he remembered our conversation.

I walked into the kitchen to wash the banana off the knife and heard him say something. I couldn't understand him because he was so soft-spoken, so rather than try to talk and listen over the running water, I waited until I was done with the knife. I planned to ask him what he had said but I knew I ran the risk that he would already have forgotten. When I turned off the water, Dad said, "Did you hear what I said?" Another amazement. He knew the sound of the water had made it difficult for me to hear him. I said I hadn't but that I wanted to know what he said. Dad responded, "The Lord wants me to care. That's it. He wants me to care." I said, "Daddy, He knows you care. I think right now, what you care about most is seeing Him." He cried some more. We both did.

I prayed that the little verse box that sat on their table would be a means of grace that morning, but when Mama pulled the verse out before breakfast, it wasn't anything "special" to the situation. Then she asked the blessing. Part of her prayer was, ". . . thank you for the night's rest and for Your care." I was stopped in my tracks. She had a hard time finishing because of her tears. Daddy cried, too, and so did I. Before I left, I put my arm around Dad and said, "You know . . . we were talking about the Lord caring. Did you hear Mama pray and give thanks for His care? That was an act of faith and a testimony." What a mercy from God on that hard morning. Mom had been unaware of our conversation but God had not.

Grandchildren's Care

Two grandchildren lived with Mom and Dad during some of the hard Alzheimer's days. Sara, a granddaughter and a freshman at a local university moved in with them in January of 2004 to give Grandmamma some company at night. When she went home for the summer, our son, Kenny, a junior in college, moved in with them. When Sara came back to town for the fall semester, she and Kenny both stayed with Mom and Dad to provide moral support and help wherever they could. Late in this time frame, Mom sent the following email to me.

Just between you and me I want to tell you what a special boy you have. My back hurt the worst yesterday it's ever hurt in my whole life. I started doing the supper dishes (over his [Ken's] protests) while he was still eating because I thought he'd had enough to deal with [his truck was broken down]. Granddaddy had been real obstinate during our supper (the front moving in, I'm sure). I finally gave up on one of his pills (it was a little one, too) after he spit it out the third time. I'm afraid I had given up being cajoling and sweet (but I was for a long time). Kenny sat down and was SO sweet with him. Finally I had to give up on the dishes and go lay down. Daddy came back and wanted to know what he could do to help. I told him the best help he could give was to be sweet and cooperative for whoever helped him get ready for bed. He said Okay. Kenny came back and got him all ready and in bed and Daddy was cooperative. I told him what a big help he'd been. Then Kenny said, "Let's pray." He prayed the sweetest prayer . . . not just a bunch of memorized clichés. He asked the Lord to please help me because

my back was hurting. Then he asked the Lord to please help his
truck because it was hurting, too. That was just a small part of
it. I thought his mama and daddy ought to know. Thank you for
such a fine grandson that I'm so proud of.

We were blessed to have young adult children/grandchildren who waged war with us against Alzheimer's.

Beautiful Dreamer

Mom and Dad were being crushed with the burden of Alzheimer's. Daddy hallucinated and slept less and less at night. Some mornings I could hardly keep him moving when it was time to get dressed. Mama dealt with it all, the nonsense talk and his seeing things that weren't there. She was exhausted mentally and physically but not able to get any sleep.

Never mind that Dad still had Alzheimer's and had lost so much ground in the year since I had been coming to dress him. The morning was still better. It took forever to get him up, and I almost despaired. But once he got up, things improved ever so slightly. He laughed a little and he whistled some. He whistled Beautiful Dreamer. Normally Daddy whistles hymns, but for some reason this morning his mind wandered back to memories of a song that had been played and heard many times in our house. When he ran out of whistle, I said, "Daddy, that was beautiful." He said, "It was? What was it?" I said, "It was *Beautiful Dreamer* and it was just beautiful."

Not only did he act better, but he looked better too, sitting on the side of the bed in a new pair of blue jeans. His head was up and his eyes were open as opposed to his head bowed down with his eyes closed like he did so often. I wanted this memory to be forever imprinted in my mind. I can still see him today, sitting there on the side of the bed in his new blue jeans. Miss you, Dad.

A Year's Decline

Mornings became a struggle to get him dressed. He wanted to stay in bed. One morning in February, he would not get up. I couldn't tell if he was asleep or pretending to be asleep because his eyelids moved even though his breathing was deep and steady. Regardless of which was true, he didn't get up and I had to go on to work.

There was nothing that made me feel better except "we won't stay here."

Another morning in February, both Mama and Daddy were awake when I got there. Dad had been up several times during the night. Exhausted, Mom would wake up when he would come back to bed. Finally, one time she woke up but he was not in bed. She called Kenny to help because her back hurt so badly, she knew she couldn't manage by herself. Daddy was sitting in the Captain's Chair by the kitchen table. Kenny managed to get him back to bed.

In the morning, in spite of little sleep, Daddy seemed alert compared to the last two weeks. It wasn't long, though, before I realized he may have been more awake, but he was further away from me and the present than ever before. Not only did he not know who I was, which all of us had seen at some point, he wasn't even glad to see me. He was uncomfortable around me, kept his head turned to the side, and was reluctant about everything I asked him to do. It was obvious the longer he was up, the more overwhelmed he became. He started out wide-eyed but within a half-hour he was sitting with eyes closed like he was trying to shut out all distractions and manage life one second at a time. About half-way through getting dressed, he leaned over and hugged me, which was one of those roses among the thorns.

As for getting dressed, Ken had told me to physically show him what I wanted him to do. That information was a God-send. I couldn't get his left arm in his long john shirt. I finally stood in front of him with my back to him and put my arm behind my back. I said, "Daddy, I need you to put your arm behind your back like this" and he did. It didn't completely conquer the situation because I had a time getting his arm back in front, but that technique did at least produce some good results. Besides the emotional stab in the heart of watching him, my biggest concern that morning was the struggle he went through trying to transfer his weight from one leg to the other in order to get in the shower. I was sure he was going to fall because he was trying to move forward with the wrong leg.

We didn't get in the bathroom to shave until 8:20. I almost handed him the razor and left for work because of the time. When I bent down to throw away a Kleenex and stood back up to go, he was shaving his face with the side of the razor. It broke my heart. I said, "Here Daddy. Let me help you. We'll get it all cleaned up so you're good to go." I got him shaved, and then noticed his hair. It was messed up. I picked up the comb and said, "Oh one more thing. I want to comb your hair so you're all dressed." I combed with quick strokes, but not hard ones. When I laid the comb down, I said, "We're all done, Daddy." He said, "I'm sorry. That . . . felt so good. I enjoyed that." I said, "You know what? I enjoyed it, too. That's why even though I'm very late to work, I don't care." He laid his head ever so gently on my shoulder, and I cried.

I said, "Let's go on out to the kitchen and get some juice, some hot water, and some cereal." Then I flipped on lights as I walked so the atmosphere was inviting rather than making him step from a lit room to a semi-dark one.

I got the juice to the table as he was getting there. He was more distant and yet he sat down easier than he'd done in a long time. I handed him the juice but all he did was keep leaning his head forward until I thought it would end up on the table. I believe it would have if I hadn't realized he was trying to get to the glass with his mouth. After exchanging a taller glass for the short one and adding a straw, we made progress and he was able to drink. Mama was putting the cereal in the bowls, and that was how I left them. That morning was one of the hardest I'd had to deal with. I don't know why. There have been some hard mornings, but it was as if multiple pieces of Daddy were gone forever.

In a year's time, I never thought I'd see Dad not get up at all. One morning, I arrived at work a little earlier than I had in a long time because he wouldn't get up. That was where we were in the Alzheimer's battle. This whole journey started with helping Daddy with his socks because Mama's back couldn't handle it. Then I took over the shower routine "because Mama's back couldn't handle it." Then they slept in because Daddy kept Mama up at night. I would wake them up when I got to the house. Now, after a year of mornings, I could not get Daddy up. He saw me, but from that point on he kept his eyes closed even though it required effort. I finally left before 8:00 a.m. A home health care worker was scheduled for later that morning. I prayed Mom would use her.

Hard Decisions

Our family had reached the conclusion in late March that Dad could not be cared for at home. The situation was too dangerous for Mom. Dad owned antique guns. We had taken the ammunition out of the house some time ago, but Dad was so strong, he didn't need ammunition. There were butcher knives in the kitchen. There was his brute strength. There was Mom's frailty and complete exhaustion. Heartache and hard conversations. Not everyone was in complete agreement but the decision was finally made to put him in a home for two weeks to give Mom a break. We divided up the responsibilities. Some provided the money to pay for his care. Others ferried Mom away so she didn't have to watch his things get packed up. Some stayed with Dad and packed his clothes.

He knew something was happening and he knew it had to do with him. The night his clothes and necessities were packed, he said to me through quiet tears, "Please, please . . . don't ever . . . be a-a-ashamed of me." His broken heart flowed out of eyes and nose. I sobbed. "Never in this lifetime or the next, Daddy." He did not resist during the trip to the nursing home, and while he was serious and somber, there was no self-absorbed begging for a reversal of the decision. *He was brave for all of us.*

He was there longer than two weeks, and although he did come home, he did not stay home. We had to move him permanently to a facility by early May.

There was no relief from Alzheimer's pain in a nursing home. If he were found clean, eating, or clapping to music, that was a good day. On bad days, there were black eyes, bruises up and down his arms, or filthy Depends on tender skin. Nights were nightmares.

We heard stories of him crawling up and down the hall to spy out the enemy. Like other residents, he would end up in the wrong bed. I got there early one morning and couldn't find him anywhere. Panic rose in my throat but I walked the halls calmly looking for him. He was in the last room on the hall. It was empty and dark and he had no idea why he was there or where to go from there.

These were hard things. We did what we could for him but it was never enough. Alzheimer's advanced beyond every battle we staged to prolong his life and ease his pain.

2006 — He Won

Sad Realities

Almost a year to the date that Dad had moved into the nursing home, he suffered a small stroke. Our family doctor was a gift from God. He made visits to the nursing home and checked on Dad. He recommended physical therapy that we could do to help recover some strength in Dad's left side, like massaging fingers and hand and bending/straightening his left leg. Because of a long-standing relationship with this doctor, we trusted his assessment of where we were.

Eventually, Dad was so bad off he had to be moved to a facility in another state. It was the lowest point our family experienced. Mom felt betrayed. She was unable to drive herself there so she was dependent on someone to take her and to bring her home. If she decided to stay with him, the trip required two people because the person going wasn't usually going for the night. She was frail herself, but she oversaw his care those first few days until she was satisfied the caregivers were doing their jobs well.

After about fourteen days, Dad was assessed and we were told he was in immediate danger of dying from choking or aspirating. We had two choices: 1) insert a feeding tube, or 2) continue nourishment with the risk of sudden death. The family agreed to bring Dad home and devote ourselves to caring for him and Mom the best we could.

Daddy came home Tuesday, August 22, 2006. Warren and Ken put a mattress in the back of Warren's van and drove to North Carolina to get him. After the trip home, when they unloaded Dad from the van, Warren leaned over and whispered, "Dad, you're home." Daddy's response? "Praise the Lord." I do not know the last time he had communicated on purpose. He knew he was home and he was thankful. What a sweet memory and testimony during a bittersweet time.

Home

Hospice counseled no more liquids or food. Dad was trying to die and we were prolonging it. What a relief and what a day if Dad were to go home! "The righteous who walks in his integrity — blessed are his children after him!" [19] Amen to that! With confidence, I could say Daddy was just because the righteousness of Christ was applied to him. There were no questions about Dad's character although this did not save him.

We his children were reaping an inheritance far richer than silver or gold or medals bestowed by his country. He served all: he served in every aspect of life. Spiritually, he led a flock and constantly looked for individuals with which to share the gospel. Emotionally, he had one of the most joyful hearts I know and yet he sorrowed with those who sorrowed. Physically, he would go anywhere, do anything, fix anything for people in need. He did all this not to earn his justification but because he loved God who had justified him for all eternity. None of it was manufactured or fake. He lived a I Corinthians 13 life toward God and man.

I never heard Daddy question God or speak evil of Him. And it wasn't his custom to do that with man, made in God's image. He was patient, enduring to the end, longsuffering even in his praise. When he could no longer talk, he tried to hum. How was this kind of life possible? He saw a Savior on a cross for all his sins. He saw the perfect law-fulfilling life of that Savior applied to him. Dad believed that Christ was made sin for him that he, Dad, might be made the righteousness of God in Christ. He saw an empty tomb. He saw by faith a risen victorious Savior standing at the right hand

---

[19] Proverbs 20:7.

of God, interceding for him and welcoming him home. Christ made this life and lifestyle possible. This was the blessing that belonged to his children.

Daddy entered the presence of God on Sunday, August 27, 2006, about 4:20 p.m. I was surprised at the sadness when he passed. Surely it was because he looked so pitiful lying there as we gathered around him. Pitiful because he was dead, and pitiful because of a diseased body. But this pitifulness was not his reality *at that very moment.* He left us but he was immediately in the presence of God, in a real place with real people, including his real Savior, the Lord Jesus Christ.

On July 7, 1945, The Armored Attacker wrote this about Dad:

> "T/Sgt. Horace W. Lennon is a quiet, unassuming soldier, but his actions have spoken much louder than do his words. High acclaim was bestowed on this Acting First Sergeant of Co. A of the 25th Armd. Engr. Bn., recently when Maj. Gen. Robert W. Grow presented him with a special wrist watch, one of two such gifts issued in the VIII Corps. (The second was given to a 30th Inf. Dev. soldier.)
>
> The presentation ceremony was conducted in Gen. Grow's office in the Division CP in Apolda, and was witnessed by Lt. Col. Philip H. Pope, Washington, D. C., Chief of Staff, and Lt. Col. Donald C. Williams, Kansas City, Mo., 25th Engr. Bn. CO.
>
> Sgt. Lennon, who hails from Delco, N. C., has been named as one of the top notch fighting men in the Division. Each of the commands within the Super Sixth selected an outstanding man from their respective units, and from this group of five names the winner was chosen.
>
> The watch, which contains a series of dials, tells, among other things, the day, date, and month of the year. Mileage can be computed, and it is also equipped as a stop watch.

The 26-year-old Carolina soldier, who during the nine month campaign was Platoon Sergeant, has been thrice decorated. He received the Bronze Star Medal, the Silver Star Medal, and the oak leaf cluster to the Silver Star Medal. [Dad's other medal was awarded after this article.]

The citation accompanying the cluster to the Silver Star stated in part: 'He has displayed the highest type of gallantry and leadership by his personal efforts in laying and removing mines in the path of advancing and withdrawing troops, despite enemy fire and extremely cold weather. In the vicinity of Arloncourt and Bizory, Belgium, he personally led his men in the task of marking extremely hazardous enemy minefields. On 14 January 1945 at Margaret, Belgium, he organized and led his squad of engineers in assisting the infantry to clear out the remaining enemy in the town.'

Lennon entered the service on March 21, 1942 at Ft. Bragg, N. C. and arrived at Camp Chaffee, Ark., on April 1, 1942, where he joined the 6th Armored Division. He has been a member ever since. He is the son of Mr. and Mrs. Q. M. Lennon, of Route 1, Delco." [20]

His battle with Alzheimer's was his greatest fight. Like the Armored Attacker, I have recorded his character, his valor, and his faith. His life and testimony under great duress is our heritage. His praise in spite of suffering, our teacher. His steadfastness to the end, our example. For those who only know him through this book, he truly was a "most worthy, deserving soldier."

---

[20]   6th Armored Division, Armored Attacker, 7 Jul 1945.